The Health Detective's Handbook

The Health Detective's Handbook

A Guide to the Investigation of Environmental Health Hazards by Nonprofessionals

edited by Marvin S. Legator,
Barbara L. Harper, and Michael J. Scott

The Johns Hopkins University Press
Baltimore & London

The Johns Hopkins University Press, 701 West 40th Street,
Baltimore, Maryland 21211
The Johns Hopkins Press Ltd, London

The paper in this book is acid-free and meets the guidelines for
permanence and durability of the Committee on Production
Guidelines for Book Longevity of the Council on Library Resources.

Library of Congress Cataloging in Publication Data
Main entry under title:

The Health detective's handbook.

    Bibliography: p.
    Includes index.
    1. Epidemiology—Popular works. 2. Health surveys—
Citizen participation. 3. Environmental health—Citizen partici-
pation. 4. Health education. I. Legator, Marvin S., 1926-
II. Harper, Barbara L. III. Scott, Michael J. [DNLM: 1. Con-
sumer Participation—methods—handbooks. 2. Environmental
Pollution—prevention & control—handbooks. 3. Epidemiologic
Methods—handbooks. 4. Health Surveys—handbooks.
WA 39 H434]
RA653.H43 1985   363.1   84-20105
ISBN 0-8018-2444-3 (alk. paper)
ISBN 0-8018-2466-4 (pbk. : alk. paper)

Contents

Figures

vii

Tables

ix

Introduction

Marvin S. Legator
Barbara L. Harper

he study of the various factors that determine how often, in how many people, and in which particular people disease occurs is called epidemiology. Two general kinds of studies are done: "descriptive" and "analytical." This manual will guide you step by step through a "descriptive" study of the overall health of members of your community, geared toward environmental issues. We believe there are usually enough resources within the community itself, in terms of time, energy, common sense, and intelligence, that a high-quality general health survey can be done at the local level. You should be able to conclude either that there are no adverse health effects owing to toxic substances or that there really is an increase in diseases or conditions that could be related to toxic substances. The actual determination of the cause of the health effects or the source of contamination and a rigorous confirmation of the extent of the problem fall under the heading of "analytical" studies, which are beyond the scope of this manual. Your local survey, however, should be enough to convince local or state officials that your situation deserves an in-depth analytical study (fig. I.1).

We have organized the manual into sections on background information (chapters 1–5), practical guidelines (chapters 6–7), sources of assistance and pathways of legal recourse (chapters 8–9), and resources (chapter 10). We have put the guidelines after what may seem an overwhelming amount of background material

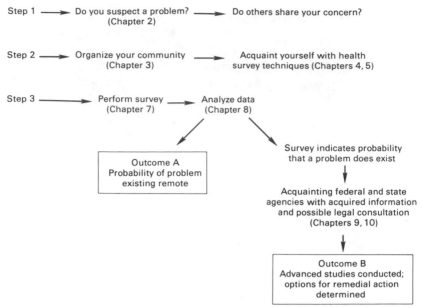

Figure I.1   Flow Chart: Steps in the Investigation of Health
Hazards

so that one will not go charging off to slay dragons without knowing what to do and why and how to do it. Since so many possible
situations can arise around environmental issues, reading the background material is absolutely necessary so you can pick out items
that are particularly relevant to your local situation. For instance,
an airborne pollutant from an industrial complex might warrant
use of a certain method of correlating distance from the complex,
wind direction, and symptoms. On the other hand, a community
evenly exposed to water contaminants requires a different approach.
After a thoughtful consideration of the kind of survey that would
be appropriate to your situation and the specific answers you are
looking for, you should be able to proceed smoothly through the
second section.

Part 2 contains practical suggestions on how to proceed. Chapter
6 furnishes a questionnaire you can use; it explains every question
included and indicates which ones are essential and which are
optional. This chapter also includes instructions for tabulating the
answers; the following chapter deals with statistical issues.

Part 3 describes the steps to take if you have concluded that an
adverse health effect exists. These are "analytical" steps such as

verification, or confirmation that the problem is real, determining causality, and investigating some of the other possible factors that were not included in the general health survey. You may want to do some of this yourselves, but the more likely function of your group at this point is to learn what needs to be done by professional epidemiologists and get them to do it. Chapter 9 describes some of the legal implications of each kind of survey (descriptive and analytical) and in particular discusses some of the problems unique to proving a cause for chronic diseases such as cancer, which is a complex process that takes many years to develop.

We have tried to write so we can be understood by an intelligent person with a high-school education or by a person who has had some college education but not in the biological sciences. We recommend using a medical dictionary, particularly for terms relating to health effects or diseases, but most actual diseases are given by name only and not by detailed description to avoid self-diagnosis by the general reader.

The need for a manual on environmental investigation for non-professionals has become apparent as communities have sought help to investigate perceived health problems. In some instances citizens in neighborhoods close to industrial sites, such as petrochemical plants or waste disposal areas, have become concerned about the risk these sites represent to the health of their families. In other instances members of a community have become aware that several of their neighbors were affected by the same illness. In almost all cases, the concerned citizens have been frustrated in their attempts to interest local or state agencies in assisting them. Limited budgets and lack of resources restrict the ability of government agencies to respond to such concerns except in the most extreme circumstances, and so insidious problems such as a rise in cancer rates or adverse effects on reproduction may not be given a high priority for investigation, whereas an acute problem such as an infectious disease demands attention.

The situation in the small community of Palestine, Texas, is a good example. An investigative reporter was impressed by the number of brain tumors among children in her community. After satisfying herself that the total number was indeed disproportionate, she wrote an article for the local newspaper. After publication of her story, she approached the Texas State Department of Health to ask for an investigation. Because of budgetary constraints, however, they were unable to assist the community in evaluating the extent of the problem or even to determine if a problem did exist. They were able only to furnish statewide data on the incidence of brain tumors and to suggest, on the basis of these data, that a problem might exist. Without a thorough epidemiologic survey, the findings of the investigative reporter might have been only a chance observation. On the other hand, the children (and the adults) in her community might well be at increased risk of developing brain tumors, various malignant tumors, or other health problems. The reporter's observation would not justify an agency to undertake an epidemiologic study costing thousands of dollars. So nothing will be done in Palestine, not because the concerned agencies are not interested, but simply because they do not have enough skilled professionals to investigate every such report with a full-scale epidemiologic study.

One of the difficulties in an epidemiologic study that is searching for chronic effects as well as for acute but subtle or vague effects is that the data can be accumulated only after a significant number of persons are affected. Such studies therefore must be begun as early as possible to minimize the number of victims and to permit remedial action.

One might well ask, How great is this problem? How many communities are in need of studies that are not being done? The Environmental Protection Agency (EPA) estimates that up to fifty thousand hazardous waste sites may exist in the United States, that 90 percent of these potentially pose a health threat because they are improperly located or poorly managed, and that two thousand are currently threatening the health of nearby communities (Hart 1978). Thus the hazardous waste problem is large not only because of the number of sites but also because these sites are usually close to the places where people live and work (Paigen 1982). In addition, chemical sprays, used heavily in certain areas, further increase the background of chemical products in the environment. The need to identify potential adverse effects from all these sources is paramount.

Is there an alternative to traditional epidemiologic studies? Can a meaningful data base be generated without the costly traditional approach to community studies? We believe that such an alternative approach exists. Motivated citizens, given the proper guidance, can generate meaningful data. They can, with professional support, determine the probability that a problem is present. The goal of this manual is to provide guidelines to permit citizens to pursue such a study on their own. Epidemiology is a labor-intensive field. The motivated members of a community, who believe they may have a problem, are in the best position to ensure that the needed hours of labor are given to the project.

The alternative approach to traditional epidemiologic study presented here offers a practical way for laypersons to proceed. If you follow the step-by-step method outlined, you can expect to accumulate a data base to present to state and local agencies in support of a request for further action. The manual is written in simple language. We make the assumption that our readers are totally ignorant of this area of investigation but, given the proper tools, can develop the necessary information in a professional manner.

Part 1

Background Information

1   You Can Do It Too
Identification of Health Hazards by Nonprofessionals

Marvin S. Legator

rofessionals in any scientific field, whose expertise stems from years of specialized training, often give the impression that what they do and understand is unique to their calling. They write scholarly articles for journals aimed at a professional audience, they give lectures to colleagues that are intended to express and re-fine the complexities of their discipline, and they develop highly analytical skills in criticizing their own work and the work of others. As a consequence their techniques, and even their terminology, may seem incomprehensible to the uninitiated.

I do not wish to minimize the importance of refined and special-ized knowledge. An epidemiologist, for example, must be familiar with experimental design, sampling techniques, statistical methods, and the biology of organisms. I do suggest, however, that trained professionals do not have exclusive rights to their areas of investi-gation and that untrained people can, in fact, perform early, simple epidemiologic studies that will be as sound as those performed by professionals and that certainly will not compromise the scientific integrity of later investigations by professionals.

In discussing the myth of exclusivity that is so pervasive in the scientific world, I am reminded of an episode that occurred while I was a branch chief with the Food and Drug Administration in Washington, D.C. Our office was involved in research on a toxic

3

substance produced by a mold that grows on various crops, especially nuts. I thought our research would be expedited if someone from our office could learn to detect this toxin in various food products. Since analytical chemists at the Food and Drug Administration had developed a sensitive method for doing this—a chemical assay—I asked the chief chemist if they could teach the technique to a member of my staff. The chief chemist agreed to train someone, provided the trainee was a senior organic chemist who could devote at least three weeks to learning the procedure.

Unfortunately I did not have a senior organic chemist that I could spare for three weeks, or any senior scientist who could be reassigned for that length of time. I did, however, have an extremely intelligent laboratory helper. I had always been amazed at Mary's intelligence and was convinced that if she had had the proper education she would have been an excellent scientist. So I asked Mary to put on her lab coat, go to work with the chief FDA chemist, and do her best to learn to perform the assay.

Two weeks later the FDA chemist called to say that Mary was one of the brightest chemists he had ever worked with and that she was qualified to perform the assay after only ten days of instruction. To this day I have never had the courage to tell him that the senior organic chemist who learned the assay in record time was my laboratory helper.

I have often been impressed by the speed with which a layperson can comprehend scientific procedures and principles, and I have become convinced that a person of average intelligence can carry on a community survey and collect epidemiologic data that will stand up to scientific scrutiny. The methods outlined in this manual are based upon this assumption. In fact, the first investigations into the toxic effects of many chemicals have been conducted by workers who were not epidemiologists—in many instances, not even scientists. An epidemiologist at the National Cancer Institute has published an article that documents the discoveries of human teratogens, carcinogens, and mutagens by nonepidemiologists (Miller 1978). The following cases demonstrate specific methods that have been used by nonepidemiologists to investigate the health hazards of certain chemicals.

Thalidomide
Thalidomide, marketed in the early 1960s as a tranquilizer and antinausea medication, is now known to produce limb reduction

deformities (phocomelia) in the fetus when taken by a woman at an early stage of pregnancy. This side effect became known when an Australian obstetrician, Dr. McBride, observed that within a short period three of his patients who had received the drug during early pregnancy gave birth to infants with phocomelia. Dr. McBride, who had never before seen this deformity in his practice, eventually attributed it to the thalidomide. Later another investigator conducted more extensive studies that confirmed McBride's findings (Oakley 1975).

The Thalidomide Lesson

In this case, simple observation of a rare defect that occurred after exposure to a chemical prevented a far greater tragedy than did occur. Most of the time, however, the toxic compounds we attempt to identify do not cause rare defects, but only add to a high background rate of specific cancers, birth defects, or other diseases and are therefore more difficult to identify. The more common the disease, the more difficult it is to show that a specific agent increases its rate of occurrence. In most cases we have to study a population close to a suspected toxic source (a landfill or a petrochemical plant, for instance) to determine if the rate of a disease known to be caused by a toxic chemical is higher near the source than in a population not directly exposed. Thalidomide produced such an uncommon adverse effect that only a few cases sufficed to show a cause-and-effect relation. If the effect produced by a chemical is a condition that occurs often anyway, a greater number of exposed and affected people must be studied, along with a control group, before a cause-and-effect relation can be proved.

Dibromochloropropane

Dibromochloropropane is used in agriculture to kill parasitic worms called nematodes. As early as 1956 its manufacturer, Shell Chemical Company, was aware of animal studies that indicated the chemical might harm the male reproductive system.

In July 1977 in Lathrop, California, two employees of the Occidental Chemical Company who handled dibromochloropropane happened to fall into discussion of their inability to father children. Further discussions with other employees revealed that many of the men working at the plant had the same problem. The employees requested an investigation, which found that the sperm count in men exposed to this chemical could decrease by a statistically significant amount in as little as two months (Legator 1979).

Thus the revelation that dibromochloropropane could have an adverse effect on human beings originated with neither the manufacturer (who knew the chemical had caused sterility in animals) nor with the company physicians (who were, supposedly, in the best position to detect the chemical's effect upon male employees of reproductive age), but with nonprofessionals who had themselves been affected.

The Dibromochloropropane Lesson

From the facts in this case, it is apparent that people may continue to be exposed to toxic chemicals long after those chemicals have been found to produce adverse effects in animals. Moreover, even after people have been affected by exposure to a chemical, the chemical will not necessarily be implicated as the cause of the damage. Nonprofessionals should not assume that action has already been taken on data collected on a certain chemical. In fact, relevant data may not be available, or conclusions that could be drawn from the data may not have been pursued by the professionals involved.

Union Employee Turned Cancer Detective

In 1981 the *Detroit News* announced the winners of the third annual "Michigan Citizen of the Year Award," given to people who have helped to improve the lives of the state's 92 million residents. One of the winners of the 1981 award was a thirty-seven-year-old union employee, Michael Bennett, a journeyman pipefitter at the Fisher Body Plant of General Motors in Flint, Michigan.

In 1977 Bennett began to wonder about what seemed an unusually high number of deaths from cancer among his fellow workers. For the next two years, by working with the death certificates of former employees, he compared the death rate of union workers with the national death rate for the United States population and obtained what epidemiologists call a "proportional mortality ratio." Bennett used union records to compile a master list of 225 workers who had died in a five-year period. He then examined their death certificates, developed categories for the causes of death listed there, and compared his categories with those reflected by national statistics.

Bennett made some startling discoveries. Of the 225 workers whose death certificates he examined, 82 (36.4 percent) had died of cancer; the national rate was 20 percent. Within this group of

82 workers, twice as many cases of lung cancer had occurred as would have been predicted on the basis of the national incidence. Among the white women in the group of 82, the cancer rate was three and one-half times the national rate. Although the cause of the high incidence of cancer among the employees of this plant has not been determined, the fact that a problem exists was established, and this work was performed by a person with no training in epidemiology (Howard 1981).

The Michael Bennett Lesson

In the thalidomide example, the rarity of a condition permitted a health risk to be identified. In this example, a worker suspected a common health problem on the basis of an informed hunch and then gathered data. When the data were analyzed statistically, the hunch proved correct. In analyzing the data himself, Michael Bennett demonstrated that motivated nonscientists can conduct a valid epidemiologic study.

Love Canal

The term "Love Canal" has become a symbol and rallying cry for those concerned with health problems that result from disposal of toxic waste. Since much has already been written about the case (Levine 1982), I will discuss it only briefly.

Love Canal is the name given to a rectangular sixteen-acre tract of land (which includes an abandoned canal) in the southeastern section of Niagara, New York. Hooker Electrochemical Companies, now the Hooker Chemical and Plastic Companies, admits to depositing 21,000 tons of chemical waste into the canal from 1942 to 1953. In 1953 Hooker filled the canal, covered it with dirt, and sold the land to the Niagara Board of Education for one dollar. Part of the land, a sixteen-acre tract near the abandoned canal, was sold to a real estate developer, and homes were built on it. In 1955 a school was opened near a corner of the tract.

In the late 1950s, homeowners began to complain about nauseating odors and black sludge in the area and about finding chemical burns on their children. In 1978 one homeowner, Lois Gibbs, read an article in the local newspaper about the chemicals buried at this dump site. Mrs. Gibbs wanted to withdraw her son from the school adjacent to the canal, but her request was denied. She then began to ask her neighbors about their health problems and found that an unusually high percentage of the residents of Love Canal were ill in some way. With this information to enlist support, Mrs. Gibbs founded the Love Canal Homeowners Association, which serves as a model for similar groups because of the outstanding success of its efforts.

The citizens of the community were able to focus public attention on their problem. A health survey, conducted primarily by the homeowners, corroborated the informal observations of many of the citizens of Love Canal. The New York State Department of Health then conducted an epidemiologic study, which found a high incidence of miscarriages and low-birth-weight infants in the area. On 7 August 1978 President Carter declared Love Canal to be in a state of emergency and authorized "action necessary to save many lives, protect property or to avert or lessen the threat of disaster." On 22 May 1980 he declared a second state of emergency, and on 23 May 1980 relocation of Love Canal homeowners was begun.

The Love Canal Lesson

In the previous example, Michael Bennett discovered an increase in cases of cancer in a specific population by comparing the incidence of cancer in that group with the incidence in the population of the United States as a whole. Although this type of information is valuable, it is often imprecise because many factors (geographical difference, socioeconomic status, and variations in life-style) confound direct comparison of a small population with the national population. At Love Canal, however, the community organization studied the population with respect to distance from the source of contamination. This kind of study produces the most conclusive epidemiologic data for investigations of the toxic effects of chemicals, especially when chronic disorders are involved.

Although the health survey taken by the citizens of Love Canal was criticized as unscientific, the study carried out by the New York State Health Department was also criticized. In fact, a government report implied that the Homeowners Association study, carried out by Dr. Beverly Paigen, a cancer research investigator, was as valid as that performed by epidemiologists from the New York State Department of Health. The Health Department study compared the outcomes of the pregnancies of Love Canal residents not with those of a similar group, but with general statistics reported in professional journals. Such a comparison yields imprecise data, which can be misleading. No thorough, sound epidemiologic study was ever carried out at Love Canal, but the survey conducted

9

by the citizens of the area served at least to bring its problems to the attention of various officials.

Applications

These four examples illustrate the ways health hazards from chemical exposure can come to be recognized. The first step in any process is taken when careful observation, an informed hunch, or knowledge of the presence of toxic chemicals leads someone to believe a community health problem may exist. Rarely (as in the case of thalidomide) does the observation of an unusual health problem alone suffice to establish that a particular chemical has produced the problem. In most situations we are faced not with a rare anomaly, but with an increased occurrence of a common problem, such as cancer, birth defects, or neurological disorders. Since these problems can result from a variety of factors (numerous and diverse chemicals, personal habits, and genetic susceptibility), a cause-and-effect relation between a chemical and a health problem is difficult to establish, and further investigation must be undertaken.

In some cases comparing the rate of occurrence of a health problem in a group exposed to a chemical with the rate in the population as a whole may be enough to implicate the chemical. In most cases, however, the best approach is to compare the rate of occurrence in a population believed to be at risk with the rate in an unexposed group. Formation of a strong community organization is often a prerequisite for such a study. If community leaders know how to compose questionnaires, gather data, and interpret these data, they can then take steps to determine whether a health hazard exists. The purpose of this manual is to describe these investigative tools. If the detailed approach outlined here is followed carefully, a study performed by a community should have scientific credibility.

2 Do You Suspect a Problem?
Known Exposures,
Known Effects

Barbara L. Harper

lthough many environmental health problems are caused by temporary exposures and the overt effects decline after exposure stops, this chapter stresses chronic or permanent effects (cancer, mutation, and birth defects) because these are traumatic events and because there is a definite possibility that some of these effects can be transmitted to offspring (i.e., are inherited conditions). We know that we are not yet able to detect all these effects, and we do not know the effects of long-term or low-dose effects even of chemicals known to be human carcinogens at high doses. We have all read about instances where residents are assured that a contaminated neighborhood is safe to raise children in, yet officials who come into their backyards to collect samples for analysis wear protective outfits resembling space suits. Since it is wiser to err on the side of caution, this manual lists known human carcinogens (causing cancer) and teratogens (causing birth defects and other adverse birth outcomes).

Although acute and often reversible symptoms are generally viewed as less serious, they are often easier to measure and are much more common. Children, however, while often the most susceptible to hazardous substances, are the hardest to assess because a parent must observe the child's behavior and interpret it. A good study should reveal other high-risk or more susceptible subgroups. Many such groups we already know of: the unborn, children, the elderly, and persons with preexisting conditions who may develop environmentally triggered symptoms in whatever organ system is already affected. This idea is the basis for the concept of multiple contributory causes: many things (chemicals, infection, structural damage, and so on) contribute to the appearance of both acute and chronic disease.

While acute (and reversible) symptoms may have a theoretical threshold below which every single toxic molecule is detoxified and no overt symptoms are caused, this threshold, if it really exists, obviously can differ greatly for different people and for different organs within an individual. However, for agents such as carcinogens and mutagens that can in theory cause permanent damage if only one molecule gets to the right place in the cell, there is no threshold of safety. Additionally, there are many instances in which a toxic substance is retained in the body, accumulating until some recognizable condition (poisoning, neurological deficit, etc.) occurs. In other instances small amounts of damage remain unrepaired even after the substance is gone, so that with recurrent exposure effects may accumulate until they are noticeable. One more reason to justify expending the effort needed to conduct a good health survey is the multitude of effects toxic substances have on people. Some chemicals cause acute symptoms but have never been shown to cause cancer. Some carcinogens are relatively nontoxic, so lengthy or large exposures can be physically tolerated. Last, some substances obviously cause different symptoms in different people, so that one person may experience only acute symptoms while another may develop a chronic condition.

There are two situations in which we hope this manual will be of assistance: (1) if you live near a source of real or potential chemical or radioactive contamination or suspect there are harmful chemicals in your air or water but do not know whether they are having an adverse effect on health; (2) if you suspect that the incidence of specific diseases or general ill health in your area is too high (relative to other communities) but do not know whether the effect is "real," or statistically significant. This manual is meant to enable your community organization to conduct a systematic environmental health survey of sufficient quality either to convince yourselves that there really is no excess of health problems relative to other communities or to your area of the country, or to convince state or national officials that there probably is a real problem and that they should give priority to a more careful study of your community.

The information given here is not primarily aimed at finding specific causes of health problems, nor is it absolutely necessary that you know the specific chemicals involved, their source, or the particular way you are exposed. It is the responsibility of state agencies to identify the pollutant and to eliminate its source; but it will be much easier for them to respond to a well-organized community group that has good-quality data on health effects than to a few individuals who have collected some anecdotes.

This chapter will acquaint you in a general way with some human health outcomes influenced by exposure to toxic substances: cancer, birth defects, mutation, and acute and chronic toxicity. We will review known environmental sources of toxic chemical and radiation exposure, along with some professional surveys (epidemiologic studies) conducted around pollution point sources.

Known Health Effects of Toxic Substances

Almost every day popular articles appear in newspapers and magazines telling of some newly discovered exposure to hazardous subtances. For example, the National Clean Air Coalition reports that plants in Akron, Ohio, are legally emitting almost 600,000 pounds of the carcinogen acrylonitrile per year. The same group listed 312 carcinogen-emitting chemical plants, oil refineries, and coke ovens; Texas has more than twice as many plants (53 in all) as any other state. *Discover* magazine (March 1982) described the underground spreading of toxic chemicals into Atlantic City's public water supply. Also in March 1982, residents of the island of Oahu learned that their milk was being recalled because a routine check revealed contamination with the carcinogenic pesticide heptachlor. In December 1980 chlordane was detected in the water supply of several suburbs of Pittsburgh; chlordane is difficult to remove, but the "continuous flushing action of normal water flow will eventually eliminate" residual contamination (*Morbidity and Mortality Weekly Report* 30, 46 [1981]:571). *Mechanics Illustrated* (September 1980, p. 54) listed the "dirty dozen" worst pollutants with respect to the amount of human exposure and in terms of relative toxicity. These pollutants include arsenic, benzene, cadmium, carbon tetrachloride, chlordane, chromium, dioxin, lead, manganese, mercury, polychlorinated biphenyls (PCBs), and trichloroethylene (TCE). A significant amount of the produce in our grocery stores, particularly imported produce, has measurable levels of a variety of pesticide residues, some of which are "allowable" and some of which exceed permissible levels.

How can we possibly be aware of all our potentially hazardous chemical exposures? Obviously we are notified of only a small fraction of the hazards we are exposed to. A brief reflection will bring to mind many exposures similar to the ones listed above. Additionally, we constantly expose ourselves by choice to a multitude of potentially hazardous chemicals in cigarette smoke, insect sprays, paint strippers, weed killers, and so on, with little consideration for their poisonous nature as long as there is no immediate effect.

Every person in this country carries in body fat an average level of the pesticide DDT of ten parts per million (range 5–20 ppm; Roberts 1982; Wolff, Anderson, and Selikoff 1982), 0.1–0.6 ppm each of dieldrin and benzene hexachloride, and lesser amounts of other toxic substances (reviewed by Hayes 1975). In one study, DDT values increased from 0.0015 ppm (the national average for blood-serum DDT) to 0.0076 ppm in the population of a town downstream from a defunct DDT plant, and the amount of DDT stored in body fat increased linearly with the age of the individual. In other studies, DDT levels reached 1,000 ppm in body fat of DDT formulators (Hayes 1975). Finally, certain regions of this country have been exposed to individual agents (such as PBBs, polybrominated biphenyls), and almost all of the local or regional population there may have measurable levels of the contaminants in their tissues (Wolff, Anderson, and Selikoff 1982).

What are the effects of these chronic multiple exposures? We are aware of only the most obvious adverse health effects of some chemicals. In some cases we are aware that particular groups of people may be especially sensitive to certain compounds ("high-risk groups"). For example, the fetus is especially vulnerable to many things that may have no observable effect on the mother. Similarly, asthmatics are particularly sensitive to permissible levels of sulfur dioxide present in smog (*Science* 212:1251). Biochemical and physiological processes contributing to the general maintenance of good health are very complex. Chemicals or drugs may act at a multitude of biochemical or physical sites, disrupting or subtly altering the delicately balanced and interlocked processes that allow us to function optimally. Some chemicals are toxic in the sense that they interfere with the balance of these processes and thereby produce vague symptoms that can best be described as just not feeling well. Some chemicals interfere with specific reactions and may therefore cause specific or intense symptoms that are more easily recognized. Still other chemicals we know to specifically cause cancer or birth defects.

Since we evolved with exposure to low-level natural or "background" exposures to X radiation, ultraviolet light, carcinogens occurring naturally in plants, other natural toxins, and so on, we have developed the capacity to detoxify (to render harmless by biochemical processes) many natural compounds as well as toxic waste products generated as natural by-products of metabolism and to repair most spontaneously occurring lesions. Thus we can also detoxify many modern foreign compounds, but the levels of specific enzymes that catalyze these reactions vary from person to person and depend on the genetic makeup of the individual. That we can metabolize foreign compounds has two consequences. (1) Some of these biochemical reactions increase toxicity before the compound can be attached to other molecules and rendered inert so it can be eliminated from the body. During the short period that the chemical (or drug) is bioactive, it can attach to the large molecules in the cell, such as proteins or DNA, which in turn can cause cell damage or mutation in certain circumstances. (2) With compounds whose only effects are acute toxicity (i.e., those that do not cause mutations), a low level of the compound may be tolerated without adverse effect because the cells can detoxify a certain amount of it. The level of the compound below which no adverse effect is seen is termed the "threshold" level. The more toxic a chemical is, the lower its threshold, or the less can be tolerated. In addition, not every person can tolerate the same amount of a particular chemical, so the threshold level of effect may vary from person to person. The most sensitive individuals, then, are those at highest risk for developing symptoms.

Although we may be able to detoxify low levels of some toxic chemicals, there is no concrete evidence that we can safely tolerate even small amounts of *carcinogens* below some theoretical "threshold" of detoxification. Most damage is repaired by normal repair mechanisms, but it may take only one molecule not detoxified or one lesion not repaired to begin the process of transforming a normal cell into a malignant one. This will become clearer in the discussion of carcinogens below.

Human Carcinogens

Carcinogen—an agent that causes new, uncontrolled, and progressive growth (cancer).

Recent analyses indicate that overall cancer rates in persons under sixty-five years of age are not increasing (Doll and Peto 1981). However, other recent articles have shown that some kinds of cancer, particularly those associated with smoking and occupational exposures, are increasing, particularly in the older age groups (Davis, Bridboard, and Schneiderman 1982; Gittelsohn 1982). Whether cancer rates are increasing or decreasing is a controversial topic, complicated by arguments such as whether to examine cancer occurrence (incidence) as opposed to cancer-related deaths (mortality), what age groups to examine, whether improved treatment of cancer in younger age groups offsets increased mortality in older age groups, whether a decrease in lung cancer is following decreased incidence of smoking or use of low-tar cigarettes, and so on. It is definite, however, that several man-made chemicals cause cancer in the workplace and, by logical extension, in the general population.

Certain occupations have long been known to be associated with increased cancer risks (Hunter 1978), and other associations are still being discovered or confirmed (David, Bridboard, and Schneiderman 1982; table 2.1). Increased cancer rates generally parallel national chemical production patterns (David, Bridboard and Schneiderman 1981), but though some industrial processes associated with increased risk of cancer can be linked to specific chemical exposures, in others the agents have not been identified. Many industries use a variety of known carcinogens, and several popular books have documented this sort of exposure.

There are many other occupations, some with obvious and some with not-so-obvious exposures to known human carcinogens, that should also be considered. Workers in such occupations include pesticide formulators and applicators, farmers or ranchers who apply their own fertilizers and pesticides or work heavily treated land, and persons who handle carcinogenic drugs (pharmacists, verterinarians, nurses). Few occupations are totally free of at least sporadic or trace exposure to carcinogens.

The compounds and processes that have been identified as established or probable carcinogens for humans on the basis of sufficient evidence from epidemiological studies are shown in table 2.2. Carcinogens cause cancer within multiple organs, but substances for

Table 2.1 Occupation and Cancer: New Findings

Occupation or Industry	Site or Type of Cancer
Rubber and tire workers	Prostate, lymphatic leukemia
Paint and coating manufacture	Bowel, rectum
Petroleum industries, petrochemicals	Stomach, brain, leukemia, multiple myeloma
Welders and metal workers	Respiratory
Pressroom workers	Buccal, pharyngeal
Farmers, pesticide applicators	Soft-tissue sarcoma
Hospital workers (ethylene oxide)	Stomach, leukemia
Aluminum reduction workers	Lymphoma, lung, pancreas
Plumbers, pipefitters	Respiratory, lymphatic
Laundry, dry cleaning	Kidney, genitals
Leather workers	Bladder
Spray painters (zinc, chromates)	Lung
Automotive manufacture (casting, plating)	Lung

Source: Modified from Davis, Bridboard, and Schneiderman (1982).

which we have evidence of human carcinogenicity are usually potent and site specific, causing cancer largely within a single organ. For example, a very specific kind of cancer (mesothelioma) is caused by asbestos, although asbestos also causes cancer in the lung. The list of human carcinogens does not include some of the most important, such as cigarette smoke, since these have not yet been evaluated in the IARC program. Many other chemicals probably contribute to human cancer but have not been detected as such because their use is more limited, because they are less potent, or because they increase overall cancer levels rather than cancer at a specific site. On the other hand, not everything causes cancer, and most chemicals that have been examined in human populations have no observable effect. The drawback to this argument, however, is that relatively few chemicals have been extensively examined, and in point of fact we do not really know whether they are completely safe. We can never guarantee with complete certainty that a chemical is safe for everyone; we might have found an effect had we looked at a few more people.

A detailed discussion of the causes of cancer is too technical for this manual, and such causation is currently a topic of heated debate. Briefly, however, the development of neoplastic disease involves lesion(s) in the genetic material of the cell (the material that contains all the coded information needed to make a new human being and all the types of cells), abnormal promotion of the growth of the cell, interaction between host defense systems and the abnormal cell, and progression of the cell and its progeny through various stages of malignancy as the tumor becomes independent of normal limits on growth (fig. 2.1). Thus, multiple factors contribute to the development of cancer, many arising outside the body. There are five categories of cancer-causing factors, and though the exact contribution of each to the cancer process as a whole is very controversial, they may eventually prove to be of roughly equal importance. These categories are (1) smoking; (2) chemicals (both industrial and environmental), radiation, noise, and heat; (3) life-style, including alcohol intake, dietary fat and fiber, stress, vitamins, urban effects (such as smog), personality type, and general health habits; (4) genetics of the individual, including predisposition, first-degree relatives with cancer, repair of genetic damage, and other biochemical factors beyond our control; (5) other factors such as other exposure to drugs, pesticides, and household or hobby chemicals and interactions and synergisms between them, certain infections, background radiation, and random chance. Thus it is not unreasonable to say that most of the causes of cancer we know about are within our power to modify, or that most cancer is preventable. It will be many years before we can say why one person develops cancer while another person does not, but we are slowly beginning to understand some of the causes of cancer, and therefore ways to prevent it. It may be a by-product of this manual that additional causes of environmentally related cancer may be identified, or that we may come to understand the relative contributions of some of the factors mentioned above.

Humans are usually not exposed to high doses of individual chemicals, except in some occupational situations, so it is often difficult to pinpoint a chemical culprit or establish causation, and it is not really necessary to do so in the context of this manual. As we mentioned before, we are exposed to multiple agents that may influence each other's metabolism and effects. Other factors that we can control by choice (smoking, in particular) have been used as the legal defense of "contributory negligence"—in other words, the victim contributes by choice to his own disease. This defense has been used to unfair advantage by industry in individual cases, but large-scale epidemiologic studies are clarifying such contributory factors *not* on an individual basis, but according to popula-

Table 2.2   Chemicals, Industrial Processes, and Industries Established as Carcinogenic or Probably Carcinogenic to Humans

Acrylonitrile (2A)
Actinomycin D (2B)
Adriamycin (2B)
Aflatoxins (2A)
4-Aminobiphenyl (1)
Amitrole (2B)
Analgesic mixtures containing phenacetin (1)
Arsenic and certain arsenic compounds (1)
Asbestos (1)
Auramine, manufacture of (1)
Auramine, technical grade (2B)
Azathioprine (1)
Benzene (1)
Benzidine (1)
Benzo(a)pyrene (2A)
Benzotrichloride (2B)
Beryllium and beryllium compounds (2A)
Bis(chloroethyl)nitrosourea (BCNU) (2B)
Bis(chloromethyl)ether (1)
Boot and shoe manufacture and repair (certain operations) (1)
1,4-Butanediol dimethanesulfonate (Myleran) (1)
Cadmium and cadmium compounds (2B)
Carbon tetrachloride (2B)
Chemotherapy for lymphomas (certain combinations including MOPP) (1)
Chlorambucil (1)
Chloramphenicol (2B)
Chlornaphazine (1)
Chloroethyl cyclohexylnitrosourea (CCNU) (2B)
Chloroform (2B)
Chloromethyl methyl ether, technical grade (1)
Chlorophenols (occupational exposure to) (2B)
Chromium and certain chromium compounds (1)
Cisplatin (2B)
Conjugated estrogens (1)
Cyclophosphamide (1)
DDT (2B)
Dacarbazine (2B)

3,3'-Dichlorobenzidine (2B)
Dienestrol (2B)
Diethylstilbestrol (DES) (1)
Diethyl sulfate (2A)
3,3'-Dimethoxybenzidine (2B)
Dimethylcarbamoyl chloride (2B)
Dimethyl sulfate (2A)
1,4-Dioxane (2B)
Direct black 38, technical grade (2B)
Direct blue 6, technical grade (2B)
Direct brown 95, technical grade (2B)
Epichlorohydrin (2B)
Estradiol (2B)
Estrone (2B)
Ethinylestradiol (2B)
Ethylene dibromide (EDB) (2B)
Ethylene oxide (2B)
Ethylene thiourea (2B)
Formaldehyde gas (2B)
Furniture manufacture (1)
Hematite mining, underground (radon) (1)
Hydrazine (2B)
Isopropyl alcohol manufacture (strong-acid process) (1)
Isopropyl oils (1)
Magenta manufacture (2A)
Melphalan (1)
Mestranol (2B)
Methoxsalen with ultraviolet A therapy (PUVA) (1)
Metronidazole (2B)
Mustard gas (1)
2-Naphthylamine (1)
Nickel and certain nickel compounds (2A)
Nickel refining (1)
Nitrogen mustard (2A)
Norethisterone (2B)
Oral contraceptives, combined (2A)
Oral contraceptives, sequential (2B)
Oxymetholone (2A)
Phenacetin (2A)
Phenazopyridine (2B)
Phenoxyacetic herbicides (occupational exposure to) (2B)
Phenytoin (2B)
Polychlorinated biphenyls (PCB) (2B)
Procarbazine (2A)
Progesterone (2B)

Table 2.2 (continued)

Propylthiouracil (2B)	*o*-Toluidine (2A)
Rubber industry (certain operations)	Treosulfan (1)
(1)	Triaziquone (2B)
Soots, tars, and oils (1)	2,4,6-Trichlorophenol (2B)
Tetrachlorodibenzo-p-dioxin (TCDD)	Uracil mustard (2B)
(2B)	Vinyl chloride monomer (1)
ThioTEPA (2B)	

Note: IARC classification scheme:
Group 1: Carcinogenic to humans; sufficient evidence of a causal association
   in humans.
Group 2A: Probably carcinogenic to humans; usually, limited evidence of
   carcinogenicity to humans but sufficient evidence of carcinogenicity to experimental animals.
Group 2B: Probably carcinogenic to humans; limited or, usually, inadequate
   evidence of carcinogenicity to humans, and, usually, sufficient or
   limited evidence of carcinogenicity to experimental animals.
This classification scheme is based on strength of evidence of carcinogencity.

tion. Practically speaking, however, one can appreciate how difficult
it is to prove that *but for* exposure to chemical X, this chain
smoker would not have developed lung cancer or bladder cancer.
Legal questions like this are discussed further in chapter 9.

One point we wish to emphasize strongly is that there are few
individual *causes* of specific types of cancer, but many factors that
contribute to cancer. This is equally true of most environmental
disease conditions. Though specific "cancer genes" have recently
been identified, the disease process, which we know to be very
complex, can be said to result from cumulative insults to the
host's genetic material and to other biochemical processes. In a
simple analogy, we can regard the body as a tray full of bottles,
each labeled with the name of a disease or health condition. Each
bottle is filled little by little until one overflows and that particular disease develops. These "bottles" represent almost any sort of
adverse health condition, such as brain cancer, leukemia, neuro-
toxicity, pneumonia, chemical allergy, or birth defects. Notice
that they include acute toxicity as well as diseases that take a long
time to develop, and also diseases commonly thought of as having
a single specific cause. What fills these bottles and therefore results
in specific adverse health conditions? If a person has certain genetic
conditions (first-degree relatives with cancer, or known genetic
repair deficiencies, for example), he can be thought of as starting
with his cancer bottle partially full. A fetus may have the bottle

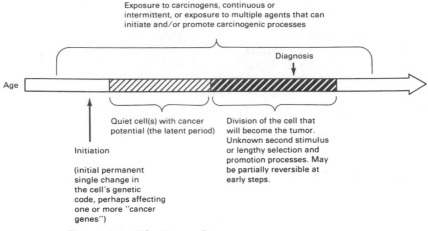

Figure 2.1   The Cancer Process

labeled liver disease half filled or three-quarters filled owing to undeveloped detoxification pathways. A chain smoker may fill his lung cancer bottle by smoking. The pneumonia bottle may be filled by the presence of the infecting organism supplemented by underlying lung damage plus an impaired immune response. The allergy-prone person, the child, the elderly person, the asthmatic, and others may all have bottles partially filled, *not* necessarily for a cancer outcome, but for other disease states as well. Thus environmental factors may hasten the onset of a condition that would inevitably have developed in that person. Some chemicals cause quite specific symptoms or diseases (asbestos is associated with a particular form of cancer and vinyl chloride monomer with an otherwise rare liver tumor, for example), but even in these situations we should not say that exposure A was the *only* cause of condition X. There are at least four reasons why this should be obvious: (1) even the rarest tumors sometimes occur without known exposure to the chemical or agent in question; (2) not all of the most heavily exposed persons develop that condition (100 percent incidence is seen only with some very potent poisons), so there must be other factors at work in the disease process; (3) although there may be key symptoms or conditions for a particular agent or chemical, no symptom is unique to a particular chemical (the closest thing to an exception is chloracne seen in chlorinated aromatic exposures); and (4) a chemical or agent may cause different symptoms in different people (a person's bottle for one disease state may be fuller to begin with than his bottle for another).

As we stated earlier, many chemicals can be detoxified, or rendered harmless, before they do any damage. At low exposure levels, a chemical (or radiation) may not damage enough molecules to cause the death of a cell, or may not kill enough cells to affect the function of an organ enough to be clinically evident. In addition, much of this type of toxicity is reversible; the damaged cell may eventually be replaced in organs that have this kind of repair capacity. In terms of the bottle analogy, this "no observable effect level" would not be exceeded until a bottle overflows. It should be apparent, however, that smaller, but quite real effects may be occurring that eventually add up to a significant body burden.

We also know of several instances where the effect is synergistic: in simple terms, if chemical 1 produces x amount of effect and chemical 2 produces y amount of the same effect, the amount "x plus y" is an additive effect and the amount "x times y" is a synergistic effect. We know of several instances of synergistic effects of multiple factors, most notably smoking with radiation, smoking with asbestos exposure, and polychemotherapy (treatment with several drugs) in cancer therapy. The reason for synergistic effects lies in the multiple effects of a single chemical or, as in smoking, for example, the effects of thousands of chemicals. Research in this area is only beginning, but it is clear that chronic exposure to low levels of multiple chemicals is a cause for concern.

There are a number of general problems with studies of human carcinogenicity, and if one of your community health problems is cancer you should be aware of them. As we have mentioned, we are exposed to a multitude of chemicals and to a multitude of factors that influence development of cancer, so it is very difficult to determine the contribution of a particular chemical. The average latency for cancer (the period between the initial exposure to the carcinogen and the development of cancer) is about five to forty years (less for some leukemias), which means it is very difficult to assess exposures so long after the fact. These and some statistical arguments that have not yet been resolved make the entire field of quantitative risk assessment difficult in human populations and almost impossible with respect to individuals. Bear in mind, however, that these arguments have no effect at all on the validity of your data; regardless of what contributed to it and who should pay for it, the cancer incidence you find is real and is easily confirmed. The scarcity of good human data and the unfortunate burden you or the state will face in proving you have been harmed by particular chemicals are scientific and legal questions that will not arise until much later and that will be the responsibility of professionals in those fields. This is addressed further in chapters 8 and 9.

Animal Carcinogens

Given the unlikelihood of detecting human carcinogens by epidemiological studies, can we rely on animal studies to indicate human cancer potential? We can examine the overlap between human and animal carcinogens. The human data on animal carcinogens are mostly incomplete and difficult to obtain (Karstadt, Bobal, and Selikoff 1981). We do not know how many animal carcinogens are also human carcinogens, but only one human carcinogen (arsenic) has not been conclusively shown to cause animal cancer, and even arsenic causes other genetic damage closely involved in the carcinogenic process. Therefore all animal carcinogens should be viewed as potential human carcinogens. Since the degree of evidence that particular substances cause cancer and the quality of experiments is highly variable, a complete list of animal carcinogens is not included here (it would include at least three hundred chemicals); this technical information can be obtained through your resource professionals. We have, however, included animal carcinogens that are *probably* human carcinogens, as judged by the International Agency for Research on Cancer (table 2.2).

There are many problems in trying to quantify human risks through animal studies. Animal bioassays are usually conducted using high exposures of a single chemical throughout the two-year average lifetime of mice and rats. This design maximizes the probability of detecting a positive effect within a manageable number of animals, but even so, for conservative statistical reasons only the most potent carcinogens are detected. Most animal studies are not designed to pick up an overall increase in nonspecific cancer, to detect early development of tumors that normally develop later in life in a particular strain of rat or mouse, to detect agents influencing growth of the tumors, or to measure changes in host resistance to the tumors. Unfortunately, people do not live in controlled environments like experimental animals, which drink pure water, breathe filtered air, eat balanced diets, do not smoke, drink, or have underlying disease, are not exposed to multiple chemicals and drugs, and are carefully bred so that we know exactly what their inherited makeup is.

For some of the more potent chemicals that cause cancer in both humans and animals, we can find similarities and differences in metabolism of the chemical, the site where the tumor occurs, and its incidence. Thus a weak human bladder carcinogen may be detected in mice as a potent liver carcinogen. Owing to specific differences in the enzymes present in various rodents used for cancer studies, a chemical may be carcinogenic in one species but totally negative in another. Other biological factors also influence the accuracy of extrapolation: latency (the time between exposure and disease), sensitivity or threshold (whether or not below certain low levels a carcinogen will cause detectable disease), and so on. Nevertheless, we should not assume that animal carcinogens are safer than known human carcinogens. If a chemical has been shown to be an animal carcinogen, we must assume it is a possible human carcinogen unless there is compelling human evidence to the contrary.

Mutagens

Mutagen—an agent that causes a permanent, transmissible change in the genetic material (DNA) or that causes visible damage in the genetic material.

Most carcinogens are mutagenic, and most mutagens, when studied extensively enough, have proved to be animal carcinogens. Structure-activity studies have given us a fairly clear picture of why some types of carcinogens are not detected in standard mutagenicity assays (Rinkus and Legator 1980). For instance, these carcinogens may act at other stages in the complex processes leading to cancer that mutagenicity assays are not designed to detect. However, once we know that a chemical is a mutagen, we can examine the role of mutation in biological processes.

Figure 2.2 shows potential effects of mutations. Some of these are well established, and for some (aging, neural dysfunction) we have suggestive but less concrete evidence at this time. Most of a chemical may be detoxified before it can cause genetic damage, most of the damage may be repaired, and most mutations, if fixed, probably have no effect. However, we have identified many of the mutational defects that cause inherited inborn errors of metabolism and other genetic diseases. We can also calculate how many of these cases represent new mutations (in the case of dom-

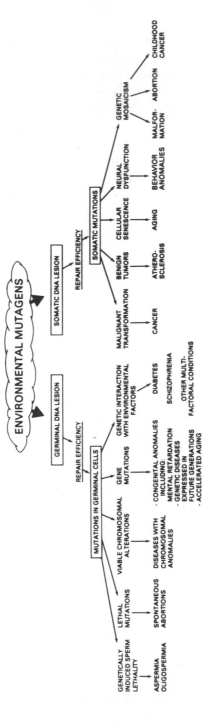

Figure 2.2 Suspected Manifestations of Mutations
Source: Adapted from Vainio, Sorsa, and Hemminki 1981.

inant inheritance), as well as how many defective genes we each carry that would be lethal if the same defect were inherited from both parents (recessive inheritance). The presence of defective genes that are not harmful as long as the paired gene is normal is called "genetic load." Thousands of diseases or conditions have clear genetic (or heritable) components and can be inherited in a relatively straightforward manner. Many others have less direct connection to individual genes and are termed multifactorial (many genes contributing to the appearance and severity of the condition). Some of these conditions tend to run in families but do not follow a simple and predictable pattern of expression. A few examples include hypertension, coronary artery disease, peptic ulcer, enteritis and colitis, breast cancer, schizophrenia and manic depression, diabetes mellitus, and diseases that cluster around certain human immune response antigens (HLA), such as rheumatoid arthritis, ankylosing spondylitis, and several others. Intelligence and neurological/behavioral conditions have genetic components. The reason for reviewing genetic disease is that any gene is theoretically susceptible to mutation, and many of these mutations may be deleterious. It is thus clear that mutation probably contributes to inherited conditions even though the effect may not become apparent until the genes responsible for them accumulate in future generations. If the mutation occurs in a cell not passed on to offspring (somatic mutation), there may be other outcomes that we are just beginning to understand and that by definition are limited to the person in which they occur. Given the multiple potential adverse effects of mutation, we should be concerned about excessive exposure to any known mutagen.

Teratogens

Teratogen—an agent or factor that produces physical defects in the developing embryo or that otherwise causes an adverse outcome at birth.

Many agents have been identified as teratogens; these include both agents that act directly at the DNA level (many carcinogens or mutagens are in this category) and others that interfere at particular stages of development (thalidomide, viral infections). As with carcinogens, only the most potent and site-specific human teratogens have been identified. Other agents, particularly drugs, may be site-specific teratogens but owing to their limited exposures, may have been associated with only a few cases of birth defects, not enough to be definitely implicated. Even if a teratogen doubles the effect of an easily recognized defect that has a normal incidence of one in a thousand births, 23,000 infants *known* to be exposed to that agent during the first trimester would need to be studied for that teratogen to be detected. And detecting agents that cause less easily recognized syndromes requires extremely large studies. An example of this is fetal alcohol syndrome, which has recently been identified after some ten thousand years of alcohol ingestion. Most human teratogen studies have been relatively large; only when a specific defect appeared, as with thalidomide, could the effect be noted in a smaller population; some of these problems are discussed by Kallen and Winberg (1979). One particular case they discuss involved the report of a slight increase in a small area of a particular defect (myelomeningocele) that first appeared in the local newspaper. An extensive study was done, but only cigarette smoking could be linked to the defect; no evidence implicated phenoxy acids, locally regarded as the obvious cause of the birth defects.

Low birth weight and prematurity are also categorized as adverse birth outcomes, as are altered sex ratios (ratio of males to females at birth), spontaneous abortions, late fetal death, and neonatal death. Known human teratogens are shown in table 2.3. Note that smoking is also included owing to the low birth weight and prematurity (and other adverse outcomes) that have been associated with it. Low birth weight and prematurity are in turn associated with problems such as poor oxygenation, intracranial hemorrhage, and a number of other medical events, so the developing brain is particularly at risk after premature births. The most common adverse birth outcomes detected in the Love Canal studies were low birth weight and spontaneous abortion.

Other fetal deaths and neonatal deaths are often associated with visible chromosomal effects. In turn, severe mental retardation has a large chromosomal component (about one-third) and an overall genetic component of one-half (i.e., one-half the cases of severe mental retardation are thought to be of genetic origin, including both visible chromosomal defects and mutations at the DNA level). One-third of the cases of mild mental retardation are thought to be of genetic origin (Blomquist, Gustavson, and Holmgren 1981). Note that "mild mental retardation" indicates an IQ of 50–69; any lesser reduction of IQ (closer to the average of 100) cannot be reliably measured in small populations. Minor neurological dysfunction of children is very complex and cannot be measured very

Table 2.3   Human Teratogens

Drugs (not a complete list)

Sex hormones (different types of DD), ovulation stimulators, hormonal pregnancy tests, androgens (cause masculinization), progesterones (heart defects), DES (adenosis, cancer)

Anticonvulsants plus the underlying disease cause a variety of effects, especially cleft lip and heart defects

Antimetabolites: folate antagonists (methotrexate, aminopterin), alkylating agents cause DD

Tranquilizers (thalidomide, diazepam, possible others) cause DD

Salicylates: LFD, ND, LBW/P, DD (conflicting data)

Warfarin: LFD, DD ("warfarin syndrome")

Heroin: SA

Alcohol—many possible effects, including fetal alcohol syndrome

Smoking—LBW/P, possibly other effects

Radiation—many effects, including cancer

Anesthetics—SA

Chemicals and trace elements (not a complete list)

Vinyl chloride monomer (DD)
Mercury (DD)
Lead (DD, growth retardation)
PCB (LBW/P, DD probably)
TCDD (DD)
Thallium
Fluorine (teeth)
Lithium (probable)
Copper, cadmium, nickel, manganese (possible), magnesium,
   arsenic = animal data only

Source: Adapted from A. D. Bloom, ed., *Guidelines for Studies of Human Populations Exposed to Mutagenic and Reproductive Hazards* (White Plains, N.Y.: March of Dimes Birth Defects Foundation, 1981).
Note: SA = spontaneous abortion; LFD = late fetal death; ND = neonatal death; DD = developmental disability; LBW = low birth weight; P = prematurity.

well in animals. However, behavioral toxicology in mice or rats after parental exposure to known mutagens or teratogens is contributing some useful information in this regard.

Although largely unrecognized, perhaps the most common "birth defect," mild mental retardation (and possibly minimal brain dysfunction and behavioral or learning deficits), may also be affected by in utero exposure or perhaps even by parental exposure before pregnancy. We may never be able to measure these types of effects—not only do we not know the true incidence of these conditions, we have no true control groups, since it is so hard to determine that anyone is *not* exposed to many of these things. Furthermore, postnatal conditions ("nurture") also influence these conditions. We wish to emphasize the exceptional vulnerability of the developing nervous system to toxic substances.

Some professionals in this field also consider childhood malignancy, genetic diseases that manifest themselves in adolescence or adulthood, and inborn errors of metabolism to belong to the general category of birth defects. In this sense we could also expand our definition to include any deleterious mutation occurring in germinal cells and present at birth, even though their effects may be too subtle to measure. This might include any of the outcomes shown in figure 2.2 as well as defects in enzymes that repair mutational events, factors that predispose us to cancer or other diseases, premature aging of the types that are seen to run in families, and many other possibilities.

On the other hand, some birth defects are not due primarily or entirely to mutation. A survey of historical associations of congenital malformations (Wynn and Wynn 1981) has correlated birth defects appearing after World War II with malnutrition; this supports earlier reports of the same conclusion and again emphasizes the vulnerability of the developing fetus. The thalidomide epidemic is well known; one of the lessons we learned from subsequent laboratory studies was that well-fed rats showed no effects of thalidomide whereas vitamin-deficient rats were affected. The special sensitivity of the fetus to acute toxins is discussed in more detail later.

There are other effects on reproduction besides adverse birth outcomes, such as impotence, decreased fertility, and so on. Some recent examples: the nematocide dibromochloropropane (DBCP) is a strong sterilant: up to 100 percent of workers handling DBCP may be sterile. The flame retardant Tris (tris[dibromopropyl] phosphate) has been linked to decreased sperm counts and has been detected in the urine of children wearing treated sleepwear as well as in the semen of men sleeping on treated mattresses. Many drugs also have side effects of impotence and sterility.

Paternal exposures may also be involved in adverse birth outcomes, particularly in decreased fertility. Anticancer agents, alcohol, radiation, kepone, lead, DBCP, and other chemicals have all been implicated as causing damage in offspring without direct maternal or fetal exposure. Research in the area of paternal exposure is still new, but such exposure may eventually be proved to add significantly to the number of adverse birth outcomes.

Special Susceptibility of the Fetus, Children, and the Elderly

Periods of susceptibility in the fetus and in children can be understood by examining what happens at different stages of development. During the first half of pregnancy organ systems are developing, and during the second half organ functions are developing. Throughout pregnancy and during the birth process, substances given to the mother essentially move freely back and forth across the placenta (Levy 1981). Major physiological changes occur in the fetus and neonate as the child's metabolism moves toward self-sufficiency. Many organ functions are not fully developed at birth (especially the detoxification processes of the liver), and of course the brain undergoes tremendous growth during gestation and early childhood. At puberty, sex hormones start to function. Finally, organ function declines after middle age, so that the elderly are in many respects metabolically similar to infants (Lowe 1974). The developing nervous system is especially vulnerable to toxic substances, both before and after birth (Suzuki 1980), and all the neurotoxins and central nervous system depressants discussed later should be considered especially hazardous during this period. For example, assuming that the fully developed human brain contains on the order of 100 billion neurons and that no new neurons are added after birth, these neurons must be generated in the developing brain at an average rate of 250,000 per minute (Cowan 1979).

Some of the effects in offspring may be very long term. Development of cervical cancer in daughters of mothers treated with DES (diethylstilbestrol) is a well-known example. Another example is the more subtle effect of prenatal X-ray exposure: survivors of in utero exposure to atomic bomb blasts have shown significant stunting of growth and mental retardation (Meyer and Tonascia 1981).

Other Adverse Effects

Most of the adverse health effects detected will not be cancer or birth defects but will result from other mechanisms of toxicity. We cannot hope to catalog all the chronic and often subtle adverse effects of toxic substances. Acute effects of high doses of chemicals received on the job are the realm of occupational medicine. There are several excellent medical texts on this subject, such as Hunter (1978), Proctor and Hughes (1978), and Key et al. (1977). Since many industrial chemicals are legally or illegally released into the environment, occupational medicine is not necessarily limited to the workplace. It is often difficult to recognize and diagnose occupational disease, but recognizing symptoms of the "mildly intoxicated patient" is even harder.

Diagnosis of chemically caused conditions is a nebulous area, and the vagueness of the symptoms leads them to be often misdiagnosed. Pesticide poisoning, for example, may mimic brain hemorrhage, heat exhaustion, hypoglycemia, heatstroke, gastroenteritis, asthma, or pneumonia. Symptoms may include headache, irritability, nervousness, anxiety, sleeplessness, fatigue, mood changes, loss of appetite, nausea, vomiting, cramps, and so on. Finding a physician who recognizes the features that distinguish pesticide poisoning from other conditions can be a frustrating task.

Another set of conditions that are probably more widespread and even more often misdiagnosed are allergies or acute sensitivities to chemicals. This includes not only contact dermatitis, but also other manifestations diagnosed as ITP (idiopathic thrombocytopenic purpura), vasculitis, thrombophlebitis, and similar entities, which have in common symptoms of blood-vessel inflammation, coagulation disorders, and impaired immune response. Symptoms may include swelling, susceptibility to infection, recurrent spontaneous bruising or small red spots, recurrent nasal stuffiness, headache, fatigue, and a number of other things (Rea et al. 1981). Clearly, symptoms of chemical sensitivity or chemical poisoning and those of a number of other diseases overlap, and the physician must be careful not to routinely exclude chemicals as a cause. Symptoms of chronic toxicity are still a major concern to the patient, though they may not be regarded as seriously as cancer or birth defects in terms of workdays lost, medical care required, or impaired quality of life in general. We wish to emphasize that not all extra headaches or miscellaneous aches and pains are due to chemical exposure, yet the problem is obviously underrecognized and underdiagnosed.

An excellent chapter on occupational symptoms by James P. Hughes (chapter 4 in Proctor and Hughes 1978) lists effects (by organ system) and agents known to act in different ways. We will

Table 2.4   Symptoms of Chemical Poisoning (Selected Organ Systems)

Nervous system
Severe headache—carbon monoxide, nitrites, alcohols, lead compounds,
    methemoglobin formers
Drowsiness, vertigo—central nervous system depressants
Irritability, convulsions—convulsants
Behavioral changes—CNS depressants, convulsants, carbon monoxide,
    lead manganese, mercury, methyl chloride
Tremors, weakness—manganese, carbon disulfide, lead, tin, mercury, DDT,
    methylene chloride
Peripheral neuropathy—neurotoxins

Pulmonary
Pneumonitis—ammonia, chlorine, oxides, dusts, fumes
Asthma—pulmonary sensitizers
Tracheobronchitis—severe irritants

Digestive
Nausea—many chemicals, CNS depressants, cholinesterase inhibitors,
    irritants

Skin
Generalized dermatitis or dermatitis limited to exposed areas—irritants,
    sensitizers, many other chemicals

Immunologic
Allergic reactions (asthma, hay fever, abdominal cramps, allergic dermatitis,
    vascular inflammations)
Diminished response (susceptibility to infection, decreased clotting ability,
    selective decreases in particular components of the immune system causing
    imbalances)

Source: Proctor and Hughes (1978), chap. 4.

summarize symptoms involving some of the organ systems most
likely to be involved in nonoccupational exposures (table 2.4);
table 2.5 lists a few representative agents causing specific symptoms
and the total number of chemicals listed as causing each symptom
in Hughes's original tables.

As we can see by the number of agents causing vague effects, it is
often difficult to prove causality. Furthermore, we are continually
exposed to hundreds of chemicals from environmental, occupational, and household sources. Nevertheless, in most situations
carefully conducted and well-controlled studies can detect an
excess of a particular symptom or set of symptoms over the
incidence in the control group. Again, this may be done without
knowing if there is a particular chemical exposure. The point here
is that even though proving cause and effect in a medical or bio-

Table 2.5   Selected Agents Causing Specific Symptoms

Mild irritants (eyes, mucous membranes) (a total of 164 agents)
Alcohols
Phthalates
Many solvents
Chlorobenzene
Cyclohexane
Epoxy resins
Formaldehyde
Ketones
Petroleum distillates
Phenol
Styrene
Tri- and tetrachloroethylenes

Severe pulmonary irritants (66 agents)
Acrolein
Ammonia
Chlorine
Ethylene oxide
Isocyanates
Acid fumes
Anhydrides
Higher fluorides

Pulmonary sensitizers (17 agents)
Cobalt
Enzymatic detergents
Grain dust
Nickel
Wood dust
Polyvinyl chloride fumes
Some compounds that are also irritants

Methemoglobin formers (16 agents plus isomers)
Aniline and aniline derivatives
Nitrobenzene and related chemicals

Cholinesterase inhibitors (13 agents)
Insecticides: carbaryl, malathion, parathion, dichlorvos, others

Central nervous system depressants (114 agents)
Acetates, alcohols, other solvents
Benzene and substituted benzenes (cresols, xylene, styrene, toluene)
Cyclohexane and related compounds
Ethers
Ketones
Ethylene compounds
Hydrocarbons (octane, heptane, pentane, etc.)
Cleaning fluids (chloro- and fluoroethane, -ethylene, -methane, -propane)
Carbon tetrachloride
Naphtha, petroleum distillates
Oxides (ethylene, propylene)

Table 2.5 (continued)

Convulsants (33 agents)
  Pesticides (aldrin, deildrin, DDT, 2,4-D, endrin, heptachlor, lindane,
    toxaphene, etc.)
  Camphor
  Hydrazine
  Methyl iodide, bromide, chloride
  Phenol
  Nicotine
  Nitromethane
  Ethyl and methyl leads

Neurotoxins producing peripheral neuropathy (13 agents)
  Acrylamide
  Arsenic compounds
  Hexane
  Trinitrotoluene
  Lead compounds
  Mercury
  Methyl bromide
  Methylbutylketonc

Primary chemical irritants (over 230 agents plus isomers, salts)

Hemolytic and bone marrow depressants (9 agents)
  Benzene
  Naphthalene
  Dinitrophenol
  Trinitrophenol

Skin sensitizers (39 agents)
  Acids, anhydrides, ethers, isocyanates, metal dust, fumes (beryllium,
    cobalt, chromium, nickel, platinum, copper)
  Epoxy resins
  Formaldehyde
  Diamines
  Cresols
  Naphthalene
  Chloro-, nitrobenzenes
  Pyrethrum

Liver toxins (25 agents)
  Carbon tetrachloride
  Polychlorinated biphenyls
  Chloroform
  Chlorinated napthalenes
  Kepones
  Chlorinated ethane, ethylene

Source: Proctor and Hughes (1978), chap. 4.

chemical sense may require more rigorous methods than this manual is intended to provide, you should still be able to prove whether an unusual health problem exists in your community.

Epidemiologic Studies of Pollution Point Sources

Many authors have documented the extent of chemical exposures and environmental pollution. The Environmental Protection Agency (EPA) has listed over 500 dump sites that are top-priority because they are near large population centers. There are fifteen thousand more dump sites of comparable toxicity that are not near large population centers and at least an equal number not yet officially cataloged by the EPA.

If this manual serves its purpose, you may be performing an epidemiologic survey similar to many found in the technical literature. For this reason, we will briefly describe some of the more recent epidemiologic studies of environmental problems occurring around sources of environmental pollution.

Low-Level Radiation

These reports include both nuclear test sites and areas around uranium mines. Nuclear exposure at the Nevada Test Site has been blamed for sheep deaths and allegedly high cancer rates (*Science* 290(1980):1097; Stebbings and Voelz 1981), and the cases are still not settled. The Four Corners area is also experiencing adverse birth outcomes (birth defects, a difference in the male/female sex ratio at birth) that seem to be associated with the use of mine tailings in residential construction (Wiese 1981), as well as a variety of other health problems of unclear cause. Some problems with general population studies conducted around nuclear facilities are discussed by Tokuhata and Smith (1981).

Smelters

An extensive study of children living near twenty-one smelters was conducted by Landrigan and Baker (1981). Increased lead levels in blood were noted near a lead smelter, increased arsenic in urine near a copper smelter, and elevated cadmium level in blood near a zinc smelter. There are many other examples of studies done around smelters and similar point sources.

Other Point Sources

Much of the environmental exposure from factories is due to release of occupational and industrial chemicals. The Environmental Protection Agency listed twenty-one types of industries cited for excess of toxic chemicals (Sittig 1980; table 2.6); identifying such industries locally may help you decide if you are looking at a point source of pollution or a more uniform exposure. Additionally, there is a well-documented "urban effect," or slightly increased cancer incidence in cities (for example, Melton, Brian, and Williams 1980). An extensive study in an industrial area of Baltimore was reported by Matanoski et al. (1981) in which data were compiled from the 1960 and 1970 census records for census tracts around a chemical plant (with particular reference to arsenic production). Death certificates from residents in those tracts (with the reporting drawbacks inherent to death certificates) were correlated with soil samples and with crude and adjusted mortalities after hospital validation of cause of death. An increase in lung cancer was seen in males but not in females. This study points out some of the difficulties in a retrospective study but is also a good example of how these problems can be handled.

The methodology of epidemiologic studies around point sources of pollution (chemical plants, smelters, power plants, mines, and so on) is discussed in a series of papers that appeared in 1981 (Stebbings 1981; Gifford 1981; Lyon et al. 1981; Stinnet, Buffler, and Eifler 1981). Problems include estimating ground-level exposures, choosing between case controls and a cohort control (discussed in later chapters), and deciding what health outcome to measure. Since point sources often lead to air pollution and therefore inhalation exposure, respiratory indicators may be used (Lebowitz 1981), although surveillance for lung cancer clustering (Lyon et al. 1981), liver cancer clustering (Stinnett, Buffler, and Eifler 1981), or a general health effect (Stebbings 1981) may be in order. Other "markers" should also be considered, such as embryonic and fetal deaths or environmental clues (Hook 1981). Most of these professional studies were undertaken because of political pressure generated by local public concern, "even though the study could not qualify as research" and thus constituted mainly a public service (Stebbings 1981).

One last well-documented phenomenon is the existence of known regional cancer "hot spots," often including wider areas that have a high density of oil refineries, chemical plants, or other sources. Occasionally a unique local phenomenon has been found, such as the pickling process linked to esophageal cancer in northern China. Because of regional variations in the incidence of cancer, birth

**Table 2.6   Industries Cited by the Environmental Protection Agency as
Often Discharging Hazardous Chemicals**

Timber products processing
Steam electric power plants
Leather tanning and finishing
Iron and steel manufacturing
Petroleum refining
Inorganic chemicals manufacturing
Organic chemicals manufacturing
Nonferrous metals manufacturing
Paving and roofing materials
Paint and ink formulation and printing
Plastic and synthetic materials manufacturing
Pulp and paperboard mills, converted paper products
Ore mining and dressing
Coal mining
Textile mills
Car washes and laundries
Soap and detergent manufacturing
Rubber processing
Miscellaneous chemicals
Machinery and mechanical products manufacturing of any sort
Electroplating

Source: Sittig (1980).

defects, and other conditions, you must either have a local control
group or, failing that, must compare your results with the most
localized incidence rates you can obtain (discussed in later chapters). Remember, you are probably most concerned with a community incidence greater than that in surrounding communities
and less concerned with factors contributing to your regional or
state rates.

Indoor Pollution

This discussion would not be complete without mention of the
hazards recently recognized in new airtight, highly insulated homes.
It is common sense that the less exchange there is between inside
and outside air, the more slowly the indoor pollutants will be
eliminated. There are many sources of indoor pollution besides the
obvious one of cigarette smoking: gas space heaters (ozone and
carbon monoxide), insulation (formaldehyde or asbestos), furniture and plywood (formaldehyde), concrete (radon daughters),
household products (cleaning fluids, pesticides, and many other
chemicals), and crafts and hobbies (paints, paint strippers, glues,
and many other things). Several instances of contamination have

even occurred from heavy application of insecticides for termites on the ground before a foundation is poured; the fumes then slowly seep up through the slab. The last item to be mentioned here is the extremely hazardous chemicals released in even the smallest of fires; this of course may be a source of occupational exposure to firefighters.

Chemicals Identified in Drinking Water

Many chemicals have been identified in water; some are the result of "rare" accidents, and some are present more frequently. The EPA has listed 129 toxic pollutants considered hazardous enough to warrant limits on discharge into water systems from the twenty-one particular industries mentioned above (Sittig 1980; table 2.6). Treating water with activated charcoal before drinking does indeed remove many of these chemicals. You may wish to inquire about the type of water treatment your city is using and what contaminants, if any, have been identified.

The presence of organic compounds in water may be either natural or due to contamination. Natural gas or small hydrocarbons produced by fermentative bacteria may be present. Organics from sewage may inadvertently enter the water system, and street, garden, and farm runoff is an important source of particular chemicals such as pesticides or heavy metals. Other well-known instances of contamination arise from landfills, injection wells for chemical waste, illegal dumping, and so on. Many of these compounds have some toxicity by themselves, but chlorination of water greatly increases their toxicity. Adding chlorine and bromine atoms to these molecules may cause them to accumulate in nonpolar tissues (lipids, or fatty tissue), where they may persist for a lifetime. The most prominent of the identified chlorinated hydrocarbons are the trihalomethanes (THMs), including chloroform, dibromochloromethane, and dichlorobromomethane. At higher doses these compounds cause the usual set of vague symptoms: headache, dizziness, lassitude, fatigue, irritation of eyes, lungs, and skin, confusion, nervousness or irritability, insomnia or somnolence, nausea, loss of appetite, polyneuritis, and effects on other organs.

Life-style

The last source of exposure we will discuss includes not only some factors with the most impact on our total exposure, but also the ones we can most easily do something about. While we tend to get more upset when we are exposed to agents beyond our control, we forget just how much we expose ourselves by choice. If we are really concerned about our own and our children's overall health, each of these factors is important in itself.

Smoking

Bioassays in laboratory animals have identified tumor initiators, tumor promoters, and organ-specific carcinogens in tobacco and its smoke (U.S. Department of Health and Human Services 1982). Smoking also contributes to premature birth and low birth weight and also to heart disease. Its effect may be synergistic with other causes of cancer (especially asbestos). It may also be causing an increasing amount of cancer in nonsmokers by "passive" or "side-stream" exposures (Shephard 1982). Lung damage from smoking places the lung at increased risk to chemicals that can affect it.

Alcohol

Besides acute and chronic effects on the central nervous system and liver, alcohol also causes fetal alcohol syndrome and is associated with some cancers (oral cavity, esophagus), as would be expected. By causing liver damage, it places the liver, the major site of metabolism and detoxification, at increased risk to chemicals.

Dietary and Social Factors

There is no doubt that good nutrition is a deterrent to cancer and many other diseases. In particular, vitamins have come under particular attention as protecting against cancer; conversely, diets low in fiber may be associated with colon cancer. High ratios of certain dietary fats may contribute to heart disease. Obesity is correlated with many adverse effects, as is lack of regular exercise. There are other components of life-style not discussed here (personality type, intactness of family units, and other psychosocial and behavioral factors) that also have some influence on the development of disease, but they are probably less important than individual genetic and environmental factors.

Environmental Clues

Careful observation of wildlife or vegetation in your area may provide some clues to extent or type of contamination. Most of this evidence comes from common sense, but it should be carefully documented. The excellent book by Waldbott (1978) contains a chapter on this topic.

Vegetation

When evergreens are damaged on the side facing the prevailing winds, especially downwind from an industrial establishment, pollution must be suspected. Some plants are particularly susceptible to certain air pollutants. Care must be taken here to minimize observable effects due to different fertilization patterns, temperatures, winds, sunlight, water, infectious agents, and so on before reaching a conclusion. It might also be helpful to document farm yields, size of fruits, or stunting of growth compared with previous years in order to minimize the influence of variation in growth conditions. In addition to the effects of identified air pollutants, vegetation damage from herbicides should be readily apparent and may result from deliberate spraying or from application drift. County agricultural agents should be able to provide much of this information.

Animals

We are all aware that honeybees are very sensitive to certain insecticides. Check with beekeepers or with farmers who keep hives to pollinate their crops. Veterinarians should be able to identify acute poisonings of farm animals, and zoo veterinarians may be the first to note effects in sensitive zoo animals. However, it may take quite a bit of detective work to trace the source of contamination when livestock (and later humans) are affected, as was exemplified by the incident of PBB-contaminated grain in Michigan.

Contamination of wildlife has occurred many times. In some areas bird populations were greatly reduced by DDT, although they have now largely recovered. Wild ducks may have high levels of lead from lead shot and from endrin or other chemicals sprayed on remote feeding areas. Numerous reports of fish kills and damage to aquatic life have appeared in the press; regional EPA officials or fish and game officers should be of help in this regard. In one study, although about two-thirds of fish kill mortality was unknown, municipal waste accounted for about one-fourth and industrial and agricultural applications accounted for about 7 percent each (Waldbott 1978, p. 56). However, these figures do not reflect the size of individual fish kills or the areas of occurrence; more detailed information may be obtained from the EPA regional offices (listed in table 8.1). Individual instances of poisoning from an otherwise minor source continue to occur, for instance, when frustrated farmers or backyard gardeners declare all-out war on bugs.

3   You Can't Do It Alone
Community Organization

Kathleen Tiernan
Barbara L. Harper
Alice Shabecoff

Previous chapters have introduced you to toxic hazards and the concept of cause and effect. This chapter will help you understand something else about your environment: it is human, a community made up of social, emotional, and political elements. There exists a structure that you will do best to work with, not against. This structure includes a vast amount of talent, energy, and concern. Here we will present several methods of organizing communities around environmental concerns.

We will begin by helping you increase your awareness of your community and of community development, then describe steps for organizing a self-study and survey. (Later chapters will outline in detail the methods of performing the survey.) If you already have some learning or experience in these areas, you may wish to turn directly to the organizational steps.

Many methods can be used in community development. *The Health Detective's Handbook* promotes the concept that you need to research your *idea* or conduct a survey to determine the extent of a problem before organizing for legal, political, or medical action.

Several things will have happened before your concerns result in an official organization. You may have learned that you are near one of the toxic waste dumps listed by the Environmental Protection Agency or that your water, air, or soil is contaminated. You may know of particular chemicals (pesticides, for example) that are in local use. If so, you will want to determine whether any adverse health effect is occurring. If you are fortunate enough to be able to conclude from your health survey that there is no health effect, then you may wish to monitor periodically to be sure that none develops.

On the other hand, the first seed may have sprouted in your mind when you realized that there must be a reason why so many children playing in a particular area got skin rashes or had seizures, or when you connected the strange taste of your water with your chronic indigestion, or when you noticed that your local childhood leukemia parents' group was getting larger and larger, and so on. There are two main points to these examples:

1. You must voice your concerns and get others to voice theirs. You may find that you have an experience in common or have the same fears and worries.
2. Keep an open mind. Don't make it your purpose to prove that chemical X causes condition Y unless you are absolutely sure this is the case.

Some basic steps to community development are listed below. Review them and decide where you are. Ask the others who share your concern. Do they agree? This chapter assumes that you are ready with an idea (step 1) and are now in need of organizational methods.

1. Define your concern.
2. Plan how to organize. .
3. Evaluate the prior situation (self-study).
4. Evaluate the need (survey).
5. Obtain a stamp of approval.
6. Organize your communicators.
7. Create an awareness of need.
8. Obtain a commitment to action.
9. Define goals and objectives.
10. Consider alternatives.
11. Outline a plan of action.
12. Select resources.
13. Implement and evaluate.

Your role, and that of your group, will change over time, as will the way others view you. Figure 3.1 shows the progression of your

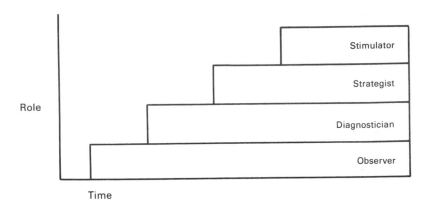

Figure 3.1. Roles of the Development Worker

role from observer to diagnostician, strategist, and finally stimula-
tor. If you step beyond your correct role, you may be viewed as
an alarmist rather than a catalyst. Do not create strategies for action
or stimulate your community before diagnosing the problem (after
the survey). You should wish to be viewed, either individually or
as a group, as friend, link, guide, technician, or catalyst; these are
positive perceptions. You may find that you have enemies by the
very nature of the problem, but there is no need to create more
enemies by misusing your role in community action.

What Is a Community?
A community is defined whenever the needs of individuals are met.
To secure a service or purchase an item, the individual may cross
a city, county, or state line and, in doing so, create new community
boundaries. Meeting health needs and solving health problems may
likewise involve neighborhood, ethnic group, city, county, or state,
or several of these. For example, water pollution may be your
problem, but the pollution source may be in another county. The
solution to this problem would have to include the organization of
several counties.

Figure 3.2 illustrates the concept that health problems can
involve populations and geographic groupings different from those
established by the usual political and geographic boundaries. Consequently, the solution community comprises the geographic
area(s) or group(s) that must be approached to solve the existing
health problems.

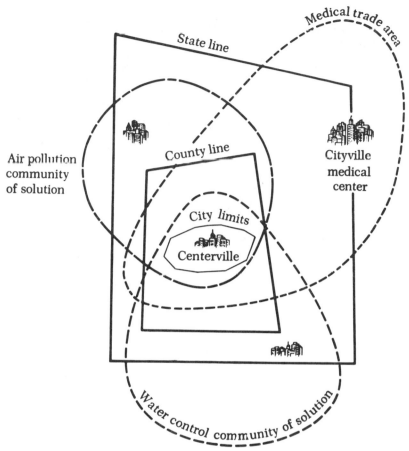

Figure 3.2   Political Boundaries versus Solution Communities
One geographical area may have many communities
of solution. Political boundaries (*solid lines*) seldom
cover all of a community's health problem or medical trade areas.
Source: National Commission on Community
Health Services (1966), p. 3.

A successful approach to problem solving starts by identifying
need. Begin your organization by asking Who shares this problem?
with little regard to geographic or political restrictions.

Gaining Awareness
Quay and Bowman (1982) promote the idea that citizens can become involved in toxic waste problems on three levels:

1. Being aware of the problem.
2. Participating in the permitting and enforcement processes.
3. Participating in law making and role defining.

Some local interest groups (such as the Sierra Club, the League of Women Voters, a toxic waste task force, a government commission or committee, or a citizens' action group) may already exist. Sometimes these groups sponsor study sessions or forums to discuss issues. There are also state and national groups. Awareness is the first step. As you become aware of local interest groups or officials who share your concern, you will be making decisions to incorporate them into your organization or to ask them to adopt your group and your problem.

In organizing for a community health issue, it is beneficial to understand how your activities fit into the existing health care system. Figure 3.3 presents four groups of activities in public health—personal care, protection, education and promotion, and social policy planning—and the support elements necessary for these activities. Your particular (or suspected) issue is usually viewed as a protective activity. Change will come by developing networks with the existing resources and related activities. You can identify these groups by starting with the yellow pages or health service directories and listing the names, telephone numbers, and addresses of people in public or private personal care services, protective activities, social policy planning, and educational and promotion activities.

Allow yourself time to become educated regarding environmental health in your community before you decide what to do about your concerns. As you are gaining awareness, you may find that other groups have done studies or surveys. This is a good time to test your comprehension of the survey technique by comparing the methods they used and the conclusions they drew with the methods and conclusions discussed in later chapters of this book. One of the existing groups may be the best one to conduct a survey on your problem. Or you may decide that, though these groups contain many resources to help you, you will organize and direct the self-study and survey yourself.

Remember, you are still an observer. You may start to form an informal group to gather information. Take the next step: conduct a self-study of your community before you organize to do any goal setting or group decision making.

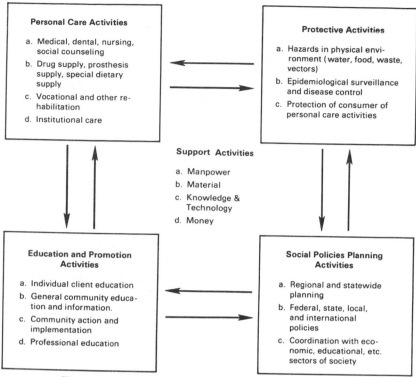

Figure 3.3   A Functional Model of a Health System
Source: Functional Model of Health Systems (1971).
Reprinted with permission.

Study Your Community

People who work in community development or planning must be knowledgeable about the social life of their communities in order to work with people and deal with change. It would be helpful either to recruit someone with this expertise or to develop a notebook on the patterns found in the social life of your community. You may begin by gaining an awareness of all the patterns, but the number of patterns specific to your concern may change. For example, details about agriculture may be central to your problem, or they may not be an issue at all. Connors (1960) outlined eleven social patterns that exist in a community:

1. Family—pattern of family and kinship.
2. Education—imparting traditional and new knowledge.
3. Government—disposition of power and authority.

4. Economy—transforming resources into goods and services needed.
5. Religion—activities by which people seek to reconcile themselves with the supernatural.
6. Recreation—patterns for relaxation in all age groups.
7. Social class—power, wealth, occupation, race.
8. Communication network—patterns of communication (personal and mass media).
9. Health—personal health and treatment of disease.
10. Agriculture—as occupation or economy.
11. Groups—critical/central for implementing programs of development; formal or informal associations.

Select the social patterns that seem closest to your concern.

Before you go off to the library or city hall to gather data, ask What am I looking for? What do I need to know? According to Connors (1960), twelve elements apply to each social pattern. For example, health and welfare will certainly be a pattern involved with your problem; you should be aware of these twelve elements about health or welfare:

1. History—objective, folk.
2. Space relations—internal (geographic, disposition of people, industry, activity), external (local, state, federal), other.
3. Resources—human, man-made, natural.
4. Technology—tools, skills, techniques to exploit environment.
5. Knowledge and beliefs.
6. Values and sentiments—ideals of the "desirable" feelings.
7. Goals and felt needs—specific concrete targets.
8. Norms—standards of what is right/wrong, good/bad, appropriate/inappropriate in social life.
9. Positions and roles—formally and informally elected offices.
10. Power, leadership, and influence—control; organizing for decision making and affecting the behavior of others.
11. Social rank—standing of person or group.
12. Sanctions—rewards and punishments that induce an individual to retain the goals and norms of the group.

Here is an example of how this study process might work. For the social pattern "groups," the twelve elements, with some study questions or ideas of what to look for, might be as follows.

1. History—number and kinds of formal and informal groups in the community; issues, personalities, and contributions of various groups; origins and past achievements.
2. Space relations—relations among groups in the community and with

those outside; distribution of membership geographically within and beyond the community.

3. Resources—plant and facilities owned and/or used by the group; financial, human, and natural resources available.
4. Technology—methods used by the group to reach its goals (formal and informal); use of professional leaders for activities.
5. Knowledge and beliefs—education of members; knowledge of the key topic of the group; sources of information used; beliefs about the group's purpose and usefulness.
6. Values and sentiments—purpose of the group and its functions; degree of group commitment; importance of belonging and participating; evaluation of one group by another; characteristics of a good or bad group member.
7. Goals and felt needs—relation of the apparent to the actual function of the group; obvious and veiled competition between and within groups; active and passive membership; plans for the future of the group and future activities of the group; aims of the group for the betterment of its members and the community.
8. Norms—standards of conduct for the members and for the group; how these norms are established; influence on expected behavior by sex, age, race, religion, social class, occupation; flexibility or rigidity of the norms.
9. Positions and roles—positions held by individuals and their duties within each group; appropriate behavior between groups; individuals who hold many memberships.
10. Power, leadership, and influence—who controls, leads, and influences each group, and how; background of these individuals; influence of the group in the community; extent of multiple memberships.
11. Social rank—of each group in the community, of members, of members within each group; attitude toward outsiders; discrimination by age, sex, education, occupation, ethnic origin, and so on of members; status symbols employed.
12. Sanctions—rewards and punishments for performance by the members and by the group in the community.

There are two times this information will be of use to you. First, it should be helpful as you organize to do your survey. Second, you can return to it when you are ready to review which elements can change to benefit your cause or to limit an environmental risk. The results of your survey should guide you to determine which elements of your community are critical to the problem.

Finally, the results of your community self-study should also guide you to several human resources. Listed below are the most common. Record names, addresses, and phone numbers as you progress. As you are gaining knowledge relating to your concern, you should get a feeling for how these different resource people may regard the problem and, consequently, how much they would be willing to help. Many of the resource people could be helpful while you are setting and implementing goals. Community resources for environmental health include:

1. Educators—teachers of science, health, and related areas; consultants in epidemiology, data-base management, accounting, or business.
2. Government—public health district officials, sanitation departments, water treatment officials, air control boards, agricultural extension service, pest control officials, Red Cross, United Way, city planning departments.
3. Health care—public health physicians, occupational health physicians, health educators, physicians in hospitals, clinics, or private practice, veterinarians, and school nurses.
4. Other groups—environmental groups, political action caucuses, League of Women Voters, labor unions, civic organizations, garden clubs, friends of the library, Mensa.
5. Business—private testing laboratories.
6. Media—exposure, expertise.
7. Space for meetings and record storage.
8. Duplicating machine, computer.
9. Other endorsement.
10. Money.

Although this manual is written primarily for groups that form because of a concern about particular adverse health effects, you may also have broader concerns and may wish to continue to address long-range issues over a considerable period. The functions of your group, from shortest to longest time frames, might include:

1. Focusing on your local problem or potential problem and determining its magnitude.
2. Conducting a community health survey and analyzing the results.
3. If a problem does exist, following through with the responsibilities you now have and approaching federal, state, and local agencies for advanced studies and remedial action.
4. Effecting long-term solutions to keep such a problem from arising again.
5. If you find that no problem exists, focusing on long-range community planning working to keep a problem from arising.

Functions 4 and 5 might involve working for legislative reform (right-to-know legislation, a state Superfund law (see chap. 8), local or state siting laws for hazardous waste, regulation of pesticide use, and so on) or establishing monitoring (air, water, and food inspections) and educational resources for the community as a whole. Directions for accomplishing these kinds of goals are beyond the scope of this manual, but information about them can be obtained from the groups listed in chapter 10.

Organization

Quotable Quotes on Community Organization

"I am a committee of one; without me there's a committee of none."

"Those with the greatest needs are usually the least able to articulate them."

"It's not what people know that motivates them to act, but how they *feel* about what they know."

"You cannot motivate others, but you can appeal to their motives."

"I'd rather my concerns die on the *line* than die on the *vine.*"

"I'd rather move a mountain than organize a committee to move it."

"If only I could type!"

"Who do I make the check out to?"

"We continued to gather to discuss problems. I quit before I ever heard about solutions."

"Who knows? They may still be meeting!"

Once you and your informal group have an idea that there is a problem (and before conducting a survey), you should take several steps toward becoming organized. According to Roberts (1979), learning experiences exist in three areas: knowledge, skills, and attitudes (as seen in fig. 3.4). The outcome of this phase of organization is a better understanding of the problem and some concrete methods to guide the group toward solving it (objectives).

Once objectives are formulated, learning must occur again. In this instance, learning centers on skills in organization, planning, and administration that enable action (as seen in fig. 3.5). Education is a key to development, action, and change.

Goal Setting

Trying to conduct a program (committee, task force) with vague or shifting targets wastes effort and resources. Working with poorly defined goals creates a "shot in the dark" approach and a mentality that leads to diffused interventions lacking impact.

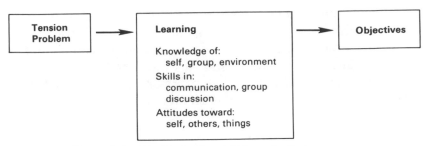

Figure 3.4   The Beginnings of Organization
Source: Roberts 1979.

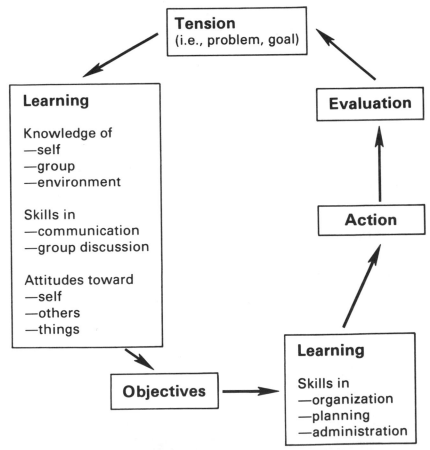

Figure 3.5   Model of the Community Development Process
Source: Roberts 1979.

Goals are statements of what you would like to accomplish. *Objectives* are statements of how you can accomplish your goals. Goal setting is a dynamic and exciting process. Be sure you have gathered the important facts (self-study) and the important people (resources). It is frustrating to try to set goals when you lack information.

Setting goals and objectives is a process of problem solving or decision making that should have a definite start and finish. Some ideas about the outcomes of problem solving are shown in figure 3.6. This is a learning process and can be accomplished at a meeting, workshop, or retreat. At the initial organizational session, you will want to spend time brainstorming each of the following topics: finance/fund raising/donations, issues and research, media/publicity, recruitment, and approaches/goals/strategies.

Preparations that can be done ahead include arranging with a local business to use a regular meeting room (with a blackboard and a place on the walls to tape up your brainstorming ideas); acquiring chalk, newsprint pads, markers, tape, name tags, and a sign-in sheet; and making up the agenda, with a copy for each person attending (Sierra Club 1981).

In addition to exploring the facts related to your problem, you need to explore attitudes toward it. Dealing in this domain of feelings with individuals (and especially with groups) requires skill. For example, some people may require reasonable standards for their environment at *reasonable* cost, others require reasonable standards at *any* cost, and yet others may split hairs on what reasonable standards are. Someone skilled in value clarification and group process is needed.

Even though one person may feel "ownership" of a particular problem, it is critical to determine whether he or she has the communication and group discussion skills necessary to lead the goal-setting process. For example, you may think water pollution is a problem. But it is not; it is a condition. What is/are the problem(s) creating pollution? Keeping the group on target and moving toward solutions is critical.

While anticipating the need to set goals, you should look for resource people in your community with the group leadership skills to facilitate this process. You may find people with group communication skills working in your community at other organizations, businesses, or local educational institutions (college or

Possible Outcomes of the Goal-Setting Process

A. Outcomes of problem solving
   1. Acceptance that there may be a problem
   2. Analysis of community situation
   3. Definition of problem and ramifications
   4. Idea selecting and prioritization
   5. Implementation and setting goals
   6. Evalution

B. Outcomes of goal setting
   1. Learn about social and economic factors in the community
   2. Document potential sources of chemical exposure
   3. Study methodological approaches
   4. Assign specific tasks for conducting a health survey
   5. Analyze and summarize information
   6. Educate community members and leaders

Figure 3.6   Possible Outcomes of the Goal-setting Process

business school). Select your facilitator carefully and meet with her or him to plan the program for goal setting.

In some cases (depending on what book you read or whom you speak to), this problem-solving process may be called "needs assessment." There are several common techniques to use. The *Delphi technique* is a method of gaining information and setting priorities through the mail. It is commonly used when people are spread out over large geographic areas. Questionnaires are mailed to concerned individuals. In the first mailing, questions center on what people feel the problem is. Respondents are asked to rank problems or set priorities. In a second mailing, questions center on possible solutions to the high-priority problems. Remember to give the group feedback The *nominal group process* is used when a group of concerned individuals can be gathered. It can take an entire day (retreat style) or several meetings to bring a group to consensus on problems and solutions.

One of the valuable outcomes of goal setting is determining goals and objectives (usually written as a position paper) and gaining some idea of the group's commitment to the next phase of learning. This phase requires skills in organizing, planning, and administration.

A golden rule of organizing states that a new organization should set itself a clearly achievable first step. This will generate good publicity, give a sense of accomplishment, and attract new members. You may want to set as goals some of the following:

- Measuring environmental health
- Documenting potential sources of chemical contamination
- Limiting transportation, storage, or disposal of hazardous waste in your community
- Educating the people in your community about the extent of chemical exposure
- Learning about local pesticide use
- Promoting alternatives to pesticides
- Investigating water quality
- Learning what your legal rights are.

Each goal will have a set of strategies to help you accomplish it. Examples of strategies for reaching the goal "measuring environmental health" include background research by subcommittees on the following:

- Fund raising and sponsorship
- Compiling a community description
- General knowledge of environmental health problems
- Listing resource individuals, groups, and agencies
- Learning your legal rights.

After background research is completed, you should be able to proceed with:

- Conducting a preliminary detailed survey
- Designing a shortened health survey of the exposed group and a control group
- Analyzing the data and writing a report
- Approaching federal, state, and local agencies
- Dealing with community trauma and remedies.

Once you have made some group decisions on what you want to do and how you plan to do it, be sure your group knows who will do what. Strive to get a commitment from people to participate as managers, consultants, or observers. Figure 3.7 shows how this may look for one of the goals. Pete will manage the first objective, and Joe will consult or help; the remaining "observers" will be kept

Goal 4: Conduct a Survey

Objectives

	Pete	Joe	Mary	Sid	etc.
1. Recruit interviewers by May	M	C	O	O	O
2. Plan the survey by April	C	C	M		
3. Raise $600 to print forms	M	O	C	C	

Figure 3.7   Assuming Roles to Implement Goals
Note: C = Consultant; M = Manager; and O = Observer.

posted on the activities of Pete and Joe, usually by reports at meetings. You should avoid having any one person assume too much responsibility, but you also should avoid asking people to do things they really do not want to do. Eventually the leader or leaders will be a source of information, contacts, inspiration, and energy. He, she, or they will make speeches, decisions, and strategies and will be creative in marshaling resources and using new approaches while being tactful enough to avoid alienating neighbors, potential volunteers, resource persons, or special interest groups (Levine 1982).

The following eight principles represent a few of the basic guidelines emerging from research in group dynamics. As you consider the move to an organization with a name, goals, and objectives, these principles may help your group survive the stresses and strains of a task like a survey.

1. If the group is to be used effectively as a medium for change, those people who are to be changed and those who are to exert influence for change must have a strong sense of belonging to the same group.
2. The more attractive the group is to its members, the greater the influence it can exert on them.
3. The more relevant the changes in attitudes, values, or behavior the group is trying to effect are to the basis of attraction to the group, the greater the chance that the changes will be made.
4. The greater the prestige of a group member in the eyes of the other members, the greater the influence he or she can expect to have.
5. Efforts to change individuals or parts of a group that, if successful, would make them deviate from the norms of the group will encounter strong resistance.

6. Strong pressure for changes in the group can be established by creating a shared perception among members of the need for change, thus making the source of pressure lie within the group.
7. Information relating to the need for change, plans for change, and consequences of change must be shared by all relevant members of the group.
8. Changes in one part of a group produce strain in related parts, which can be reduced only by eliminating the changes or by bringing about readjustments in the related parts.

There may be times when you feel frightened or frustrated with your project and the hurdles of getting organized. Be prepared to deal with public opinion and community subgroups that do not agree with you or share your concerns. You may feel that certain individuals or groups are "naturals" or "perfect" or "obligated" to share your concerns, but they may not agree. Individual perceptions and readiness to act are personal rights. You may try to enlighten people as to the threat or severity they personally share with you, but before people will act on a problem, the problem must become their own high priority and it must be convenient for them to act.

Management

At some time a concerned group of citizens must change from a group into an organization. Even the smallest component—a "block committee" or "those along the river," for example—will recognize the value of leadership roles, communication, and decision making. There will be a need to establish a board of directors, an executive director, task forces, committees, and so on. No matter how qualified the members of a group are, the group that has limited management capacity will have difficulty harnessing its capabilities.

You need a formalized management structure, regardless of the size. Select either a chairperson (volunteer) or an executive director (paid) to be in charge of day-to-day management. She or he will supervise the activities of the group and ensure accountability for its activities.

Committees

A great deal of work can be accomplished by committees. Committees enable:

- Efficient decision making
- Coordination of resources
- Systematic action.

The functions of a committee are:

- Program development—getting work done, accomplishing objectives
- Leadership training—skills, concepts, principles
- Communication—among those involved with the organization or problem
- Coordination—among committee members.

Essential components for effective committee work are:

- Well-defined objectives—planning productive meetings
- Well-defined responsibility
- Appropriate memberships
- Identifying resources of committee members—material resources, interests, authority, position
- Identifying leadership—respected, acceptable people able to conduct negotiations.

Effective committee meetings have the following goals:

- Defining the purpose of the committee
- Assigning responsibilities
- Setting an agenda
- Planning the next step
- Setting target dates
- Following up on assignments
- Making arrangements for meetings
- Sending announcements.

Agenda guidelines are:

- Call to order
- Roll call
- Minutes of previous meetings
- Old business
- Agenda items
- Individual and task force reports not included in specific agenda items
- Review of individual and task force assignments
- Evaluation.

Rules for getting more from committee meetings:

Before
1. Explore alternatives to meeting.
   - A decision by the responsible party often eliminates the need.

- A conference call may substitute for getting together.
- Postpone; consolidate the agenda with that of a later meeting.

2. Keep the participants to a minimum. Only those needed should attend.
3. Choose an appropriate time. The necessary facts and people should be available.
4. Choose an appropriate place. Accessibility of location, availability of equipment, size of the room, and so on, are all important.
5. Define the purpose clearly in your own mind before calling a meeting.
6. Distribute the agenda in advance. This helps the participants prepare— or at least forewarns them.
7. Limit the time of the meeting and the length of the agenda. Allocate a time to each subject proportional to its relative importance.

During

8. Start on time. Give warning, then do it. There is no substitute.
9. Start with and stick to the agenda. Placing the most important items at the start of the agenda ensures that only the least important will be left unfinished. "We're here to . . ." "The purpose of this meeting is . . ." "The next point to be decided is. . . ."
10. Control interruptions. Allow interruptions for emergencies only.
11. Accomplish your purpose. What was the specific purpose of the meeting—to analyze a problem, to generate creative alternatives, to arrive at a decision, to inform, to coordinate? Was it accomplished?
12. Restate conclusions and assignments to ensure agreement and to provide reinforcement or a reminder.
13. End on time.
14. Use a meeting evaluation checklist (fig. 3.8) as an occasional spot check.

After

15. Expedite the preparation of the minutes. Concise minutes should be distributed within forty-eight hours.
16. Uncompleted actions should be listed under "unfinished business" on the next meeting's agenda.
17. Make a committee inventory. Survey all committees, investigating whether their objectives have been achieved and, if not, when they can be expected to be. Abolish committees that have accomplished their purpose.

Organizational Structure

As your group progresses and you become better organized, you can consider the staff structure (volunteer and possibly professional) both to manage and to implement projects. Adopt an organizational approach that best suits the group goals and capabilities and the resources of the community. The organizational

Committee Meeting Evaluation

Yes	No	Item
_____	_____	Was the purpose of the meeting clear and well defined?
_____	_____	Was the agenda received in advance?
_____	_____	Were any materials essential for preparation also received in advance?
_____	_____	Was the agenda followed adequately?
_____	_____	Was a time allotted to each item on the agenda?
_____	_____	Did each item on the agenda have the proper priority rating?
_____	_____	Did the meeting start on time?
_____	_____	Was the total time utilized effectively?
_____	_____	Were the minutes of the previous meeting concise and accurate?
_____	_____	Were reports on previous assignments asked for?
_____	_____	Were task assignments and deadlines fixed where appropriate?

Figure 3.8   Meeting Evaluation Checklist

approach you use will influence decision making, project development, communications, and coordination. You could select a functional design, program structure, or matrix approach to organizing.

Functional design divides an organization into functional areas such as business and industry, government, or housing. Strength: each function deals directly with a particular type of client in providing services and activities such as survey or policy development for that group. Weakness: this system needs a high degree of coordination; there may be misuse of expertise.

Program structure divides the units of the organization on the basis of products, projects, or programs. In this method each unit needs to be accountable for a variety of functions. For example, a survey unit may take on the project of surveying the community and will then communicate to all areas of the community, assuming responsibility for planning community relations, and so forth. Strength: this structure fixes responsibility for all activity related to a particular program. Weakness: there may be a lack of communication; this system creates a sense of ambiguity among employees or volunteers, who may feel a greater loyalty toward their own projects than toward the group as a whole.

A *matrix approach* to management allows people to be assigned to a particular function or program but still have assignments and responsibilities elsewhere. (For example, an epidemiologist who is an excellent grant writer might be assigned primarily to analysis of the survey, in addition to writing grants for the research division.) Strength: this is an excellent use of talent. Weakness: this design requires excellent coordination; there may be confusion in reporting; demands may conflict.

These are just three ideas for management styles. There are many others. Include people with management skills to aid you in setting up your organization.

A word of caution. While there is a need for both management structure and process in a group, groups should guard against becoming overmanaged or bureaucratized, which can stifle the group by limiting the creativity and flexibility of its volunteers or employees in responding to new opportunities. Groups that do not have the appropriate structure and expertise will flounder in implementing their projects (survey, lobby, policy and procedure changes), with devastating results. The life of the group may be jeopardized and the impact lost.

Communication

One of the critical ingredients in any structure is the communication and feedback network used to measure the performance of both the workers and the overall organization. Several methods of communication are: (formal) reports, summaries, memos, letters, minutes; and (informal) phone calls, word of mouth, nonverbal acts (show of force at city council meetings). Consider the most appropriate methods before implementing plans. Formal methods are commonly used to document activities, commitments, and results. Miscommunication usually results from misusing a method of communication.

General procedures that will be necessary for reaching any goal include keeping files of media clippings, attending all relevant public meetings, exchanging information with other groups, testifying at hearings when you can, approaching and keeping in touch with political figures, budgeting carefully, and maintaining accurate records, mailing lists, and registers of residents. For this you will need space set aside somewhere for the sole use of your group; an unused office close to a meeting room in a friendly neighborhood business is ideal.

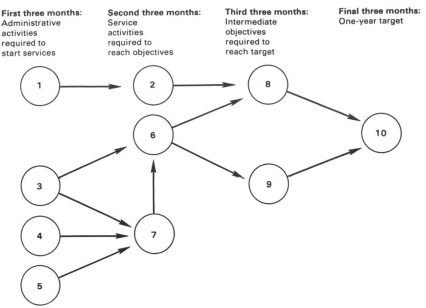

First three months: Second three months: Third three months: Final three months:
Administrative   Service   Intermediate   One-year target
activities   activities   objectives
required to   required to   required to
start services   reach objectives   reach target

Figure 3.9   An Example of a PERT Diagram
Source: Green et al. 1980.

Program Implementation

One of the most frustrating components of social action is time. It is often difficult to assess realistically how much time it takes to develop, implement, and evaluate a survey. Figure 3.9 is an example of how time may be allocated following the logic of PERT (Program Evaluation Review Technique).

First the aim of the program after a certain period of time (in this case, one year) is specified (10). Then the tasks that will achieve that end are listed (8 and 9); next the steps, procedures, or activities necessary to 8 and 9 are identified (2, 6, and 7); and so forth. The procedure is continued until one arrives at the goal or at the beginning of the new fiscal year. The chief utility of the PERT form of charting is that it helps planners set priorities and establish rough timetables for activities and makes it possible to anticipate fluctuations in resource needs. Try to get the group to set realistic deadlines with achievable goals early in the project.

Budget

The specifics of budgeting will vary according to the dimensions of the problem and the extent of the activities necessitated by the objectives. Salaries are a contribution for professional services. Salaried workers will include but are not limited to the following:

- Accountant
- Management (director)
- Secretary
- Outreach worker (survey team).

Consultation fees may cover:

- Data analysis
- Computer services
- Evaluation reporting.

Other expenses include:

- Supplies (printing, postage, office supplies)
- Office space
- Services (telephone, photocopying, data processing)
- Travel (survey travel, travel to state or national meetings).

Summary

The political, social, and economic ramifications of environmental problems can be enormously complex. This complexity can be a major barrier to possible solutions, since so many interrelated conditions have to be dealt with. Will your solutions disrupt the economic stability of your community or another one? Will they cause unemployment? What lobbyists will resist? Will every source of a problem need to be altered? Will the trade-offs and possible sacrifices be willingly accepted by the population?

This chapter has presented several methods for community development. In review, they are:

- Direct interaction with individuals and a group
- Community self-study
- Group discussion and decision-making workshop(s)
- Use of resource people
- Creation of an organization

Usually no one method will accomplish your organizational goal, but a combination should.

Consider the many "communities" that need to become involved. Individual action to fight environmental concerns is a vain hope, even at the local level. Environmental concerns must be fought on a larger scale to be effective. Public policy, supported and enforced, must be the primary focus of attack to control or prevent public problems. Individual action is best used to influence public policy and to ensure adherence to those policies once implemented. You will be ready to take these steps when you have determined the extent and nature of the problem and its solutions.

Individual action should first be aimed at organizing the survey of a situation (chapters 4, 5, 6, and 7) and then organizing to take action if need be (chapter 8).

4   What You Need to Know before You Start
Introduction to Experimental Design

Michael J. Scott

Before designing your survey you need to formulate exactly what you wish to know, so that you can choose whom to survey and what to ask them. Since you cannot survey every member of a large community, you must use some selection process that lets you survey a representative smaller group of people. You may suspect that everyone in your community is exposed equally (to evenly spread air or water pollution, for example), in which case a random sample would be appropriate. If you know of a "point source" such as a dump site, you must collect information from groups of people living progressively farther and farther away from the source. There are certain rules to ensure that the people you survey are representative of the entire group to be assessed. Since many of the health effects you wish to measure are not "reportable" and so no state or national studies have been done to determine how frequently they normally occur, selecting an unexposed community or group with which to compare the results for your own community is extremely important if you are to conclude whether a health problem exists.

This chapter is intended to give you the background information needed to understand the scope of the work you plan to undertake. When you begin a "scientific" study, you are attempting to approach a problem in a methodical way and from as many angles as possible, in order to eliminate any bias you may have brought into the study (even unknowingly). The researcher looks for the heart of the truth and tries to understand what is really happening. This process has a few universal components, so this chapter will serve as a general introduction to experimental design.

The Experimental Process

Science, as an art and a discipline, came into its own with the acceptance of four elements—classically considered to be hypothesis, methods, results, and conclusions—as the constituents of a sound inquiry. These elements, arranged in that order, provide the framework for a community health survey. Contemporary research adds another component, "analysis," which is done after the results have been obtained. Each of these elements depends on the success achieved in performing the previous one.

Hypothesis

The hypothesis is a statement of what you believe is going on, and from that stems the purpose of demonstrating that the hypothesis is correct. The hypothesis of your study needs to be stated clearly to serve as a starting point. Since you have already begun the study process with this book, you probably already have in mind a hypothesis and a purpose.

You may believe, for example, that living near a chemical dump site is causing adverse health effects in your own children. The purpose of your study, therefore, would be to determine whether the children of your community, as a whole, living near this dump site, experience a greater number of adverse health conditions than would normally be expected. Your purpose might span a wide range of possibilities—from a study limited to certain occupations to one that surveyed whole townships; from a study of a specific disease, such as brain tumor, to one as general as a search for any detectable change in health status.

Although these ranges are possible, a concept of cause and effect at the outset will guide you to select the group of people to include in the study and will indicate the nature of the problems you can expect to encounter. An axiom of epidemiologic research is that the more specific the proposed cause-and-effect relation, the easier it is to prove it exists. A paradox about hypothesis formation is that, once you have refined what you believe is happening, you actually set out to disprove the opposite. It is very difficult to "prove" a hypothesis. If you believe that living near a dump site is affecting your health, you do not try to prove that. Instead, you state that living near the dump site has no effect on your health and then set out to *disprove* this statement. This "no effect," or "null," hypothesis is the basis of the statistical analysis that will be taken up in chapter 7.

Methods

Methods are the ways you will execute the study. Most of this book is directed at presenting methods and tools to use in your work. Remember that these methods need to be *directly* useful in accomplishing your purpose. For example, a study that tries to determine the health status of a group of employees by counting the number of sick days they used in a month may be seriously flawed. Many factors contribute to workers' use of sick time, so the study may well be measuring factors other than physical health: for example, psychological health, employer/employee loyalty, workers' sense of "being needed" on the job, and so forth. Compatibility between what you wish to study and how you study it may be difficult to achieve. Try to appreciate the particular strengths of each of the methods and how they can contribute to achieving your purpose.

Results

Results are the body of information you obtain—a collection of data. Viewed carefully, they can begin to tell you something about the problem in your community. They may tell you that in a "normal" community one-third of the children have allergies, but in your community almost all the children do. From your results, you will draw conclusions about local health hazards.

Analysis

Sometimes results are not easy to interpret, and mathematical interpretation, or analysis, may be necessary. Chapter 7 will deal more thoroughly with analysis of data, but a simple example will illustrate why analysis may be necessary. If you were to flip a coin ten times and count the number of heads you got, would you expect to see five heads and five tails? How often would you expect to see ten flips of the coin yield five heads and five tails? Statistical analysis shows that only once out of every four sets of ten flips would you get five heads and five tails. Therefore, although you expect, "on the average," five heads from ten flips, in fact, at any one set of ten flips it is unlikely that you will see five heads.

Community health surveys are similar to this example in that you might expect, on the average, to see twelve cases of a certain type of tumor in your community but in fact see fifteen. Techniques of analysis can help you decide how "real" the difference between twelve and fifteen is—whether fifteen is well within the normal, expected range of tumor incidence for your community.

Conclusions

Conclusions come from pulling together all the information gathered during your study. They tend to support or disprove the original hypothesis. Since *definitive* proof or disproof, however, is actually difficult to achieve without a much more sophisticated type of effort, your conclusions will simply indicate an effect or suggest a correlation between an environmental or life-style factor and a particular disease or effect. The goal of your work is simply to provide enough basic information to demonstrate the need for further work.

The Study Design

A community health survey must be built within the framework of classical experimental design. You must define the population of people you wish to study and determine how you wish to study it. You must, by some means, compare this population with a concept of a normal group, and from this comparison you must infer the possible influence of an environmental factor on the health of the population.

Populations

The term *population* will be used to refer to the group of people being studied in a health survey. A population is simply a collection of people, though not just of the people you would like to use in the study. It is not, at least in the beginning, just your next-door neighbor or the couple down the street. Rather, it is a group selected on the basis of a specific set of conditions. If you are concerned about living near a chemical plant, then your population may be all the families living within two miles of the plant's perimeter. It must be *all* the families, not just those you happen to know. You can be more specific in your selection criteria so that your population includes only the group of people you are specifically interested in. Therefore your population might be limited to children, eight to thirteen years of age who moved into the community in the past three years and who now reside within two miles of a specific chemical plant. Since these selection criteria will determine who is in your population, they must be carefully formulated. Once you have arrived at your criteria, you must find all the children who satisfy them. If your child and the next-door neighbor's child fall into the population, they do so through a valid study design. They are part of the population because they meet the criteria you used for establishing it.

Your population, therefore, has some commonality. The people were chosen for a reason, and that reason should be pertinent to the purpose of your study. Every time you add a selection criterion for your population, you should be able to say why you feel it is important. Haphazard selection criteria can severely damage a study, either by encompassing people who are at very little risk from the suspected environmental insult or by excluding its chief victims. You should begin with the widest possible definition of the population, then add selection criteria one at a time until the final population is a reasonable and complete group of the people you expect to be affected by the environmental insult. Remember that the source of exposure and the suspected effects (such as skin allergies in children, pulmonary disease or heart attacks in older persons) are your two chief selection criteria.

Selection criteria generally fall into two areas: those that identify the exposed population and those you suspect of modifying the effect of the exposure. In selecting the criteria to identify the exposed population, you must consider three main factors: (1) Is the suspected exposure related to occupation or workplace? If so, what workers have been exposed? (2) Is the exposure geographical in nature? (That is, did the subjects live near a chemical plant or dump site? Did their residences use a certain water source? Was the community near heavily sprayed crops or woods?) (3) Is the exposure measurable in time? Events like chemical accidents or seasonal spraying might produce effects that are clearly related to time. If you understand the nature of the exposure itself, the people exposed will be easier to define.

The effect of an exposure can be expressed in many ways, so you must be alert to observe which segments of the population demonstrate extreme sensitivity to the exposure. Although the entire population may experience an exposure, for example, only people working in a particular occupation may be noticeably affected. Personal factors such as age may also tend to modify the effect of an exposure. Children, for example, are generally out-doors more and in direct contact with soil or water; in addition, they may be more sensitive to the irritating effects of contact with environmental contaminants. They may therefore be the first and most obvious group to study for adverse effects from chemical exposure.

At the other end of the spectrum, aged members of a commu-nity may be especially susceptible to lung irritants or other forms of chemical pollution. The researcher may choose to look at only these special groups or may maintain a broad definition of the population of interest and then look within it, at the end of the study, for especially susceptible subpopulations.

Other personal factors to consider would be sex, race or ethnic group, smoking, and possibly socioeconomic factors. Their possible role should be considered, though they should be incorporated into the study design only if there is good reason to believe they are influencing the expression of an adverse health effect.

Once this population is described, you will begin surveying it to determine whether some adverse health effect is present. In some circumstances this defined population may prove fairly small— because the original base of the population was small, or because the selection criteria were so specific that most of the community was excluded. On the other hand, you may well find yourself with a population that is potentially massive. Your selection criteria may not have been fine enough to identify a population of manage-able size for your study, or there may be few factors other than exposure to use in defining your population. In this case you have two basic options: sampling the larger population or adding a final selection criterion.

An example of adding a final criterion to refine a study popula-tion may be found in a hypothetical situation. If you live in a community of 25,000 amid a great variety of potential environ-mental polluters, such as chemical plants, and you think something is amiss with the general health of the community, you probably cannot be sure which of the several possible sources of exposure is responsible: air pollution, contaminated water, or occupational factors. The general health of the community seems poor, but no single age group or sex seems more susceptible than any other. Where do you go from here? It would be almost impossible to sur-vey 25,000 people. Aside from sampling (which will be discussed later), the only thing to do is apply selection criteria to define your population further.

Using occupation as a basis for selection should probably be ruled out quickly unless there is strong reason to suspect it is the source of exposure. Occupational exposures are usually plant specific (or unit specific), and the initial alert to a health problem will identify the probable source. Next, although the water source is a good candidate for the route of dissemination, exposure to it is fairly uniform throughout the community. Therefore the selection of any population will also take into account the possibility of contaminated water.

Exposure to chemical plants, on the other hand, is not equal throughout the community, although wind conditions could ensure that all residents receive *some* exposure. Combined with varying susceptibility, a community wide effect might seem to result from pollutants released at a limited source point. A proximity rule could be used in defining the population. Since the actual source of the exposure is unknown, the group of people who experience the greatest *potential* exposure should be considered, such as those who live between plants. If one area appears to be a hot spot of health problems, it can be used to guide you to the source of exposure. If you study the group with the greatest potential for exposure, you can hope to have defined the population that is receiving the chemical exposure responsible for adverse health effects.

What if this group is still too large for you to work with, say 3,000 people? If you are convinced that these 3,000 all have an equivalent risk of exposure (and thus of adverse health effects), then you can limit the group further simply by arbitrarily making it smaller. You can use boundaries such as those of census tracts, election precincts, or postal regions and by this means precisely define a smaller population to study.

Using predefined boundaries to limit the size of a population has a few disadvantages: for one, it might suggest bias in the study. The possibilities for defined boundaries are generally limited, and if a rare disease is under study, the area within the boundary will generally contain a greater proportion of the disease than occurs in the entire community. This is almost impossible to correct because the choice of boundary cannot be random. The perception that an outbreak of a disease has begun, especially a rare disease, almost precludes the use of boundary techniques to limit the study population.

Another problem with boundaries involves the reason a population is selected in the first place. You choose the population because you want to make some inference, by means of your study, regarding their health status. By reducing the population size (with this boundary technique), you reduce the population base about which the inference can be made. This means you artificially focus attention on your limited population when in fact a much larger community is affected. By thoroughly understanding the study design and communicating its significance to interested parties, however, you can use a boundary-defined population as a "red flag" for a larger community.

In general, be cautious about overselecting your population, which may create a lot of work without significantly improving the study.

Subdividing a Population

Populations are usually not uniform in their makeup and may not be uniform in their susceptibility to adverse influences on health. Individuals in a population may have different degrees of exposure to a suspected environmental pollutant or may be uniquely sensitive to it. For these reasons, we will present two additional approaches for handling populations. (These are not techniques for defining a population, which you will have already done. Rather, they are ways of handling a defined population to ensure that you will get maximum information from it.)

Generally a population is heterogeneous in character. However, in certain cases you may suspect that one segment (aged persons, for example) is more susceptible to an environmental contaminant, yet you are also concerned about the other members of the population (children, pregnant women, or families as a whole). We have already discussed how to define a population based on the group suspected of greatest susceptibility. It is possible, however, to define the whole spectrum of the community as the population, then to subdivide it—to develop subpopulations based on factors suspected of modifying a person's response to the environmental insult (age, sex, pregnancy, and so on). You can then determine who in the population as a whole experiences adverse health effects and whether certain subpopulations are more (or less) susceptible. This technique permits you to look at various correlations that might result from interaction of population characteristics with the specific environmental pollutant to yield an effect different from that in the population as a whole.

The second common technique for subdividing a population is stratification, which means partitioning a population into subgroups (each expected to be different). Stratification is especially useful if the suspected source of exposure is limited geographically (such as a chemical plant or chemical dump). The group closest to an exposure source is probably receiving the greatest exposure and should be found to have the health problems. Love Canal was a classic example of this effect: the people with homes closest to the dump site experienced the greatest problems. By dividing the population into strata, you can demonstrate the source of the problem more easily and can point to a strong association between community health status and the contaminating source. A ring system of stratification, like that used at Love Canal, is an effective technique. In this manner even a mild effect may be clearly evident among the group with highest exposure (zone 1), whereas it might not be apparent if the general population were looked at as a whole.

The choice of ring size and boundaries should be dictated by the nature of the exposure. Airborne contamination may have a blanketing effect, so that only a few (maybe two) fairly large rings would be appropriate, whereas chemicals leaching from a dump site might have a confined effect, so that the first ring would enclose the houses situated on top of a dump, the second, the houses one or two blocks away, and the third, those three or more blocks from the dump. The key in determining the size of the rings would be where you suspect you will find major changes in the degree of exposure.

Once again, stratification and developing subpopulations are not methods of defining a population but are modifications of design to take into account the specific variations in your population. These techniques should be used when you suspect that some characteristic of the population is significantly affecting the measurement of health used in the survey.

Sampling

Sampling is used to estimate various characteristics of a population without counting each member individually. It can significantly cut down the work required and still obtain an accurate measure of the characteristics of interest. You can sample a population of 2,000 people by studying only 500 of them, with the expectation that those 500 will be representative of the 2,000 as a whole. If these 500 are not a good representation of the population, however, then the conclusions you draw regarding the population as a whole are invalid. Therefore, the method you use to select the sample is important.

We can use this population of 2,000 as an example and say that your interest is recent changes in their overall health. If you send out 2,000 postcards asking these people to participate in the study and you take the first 500 acceptances, are these 500 respondents representative of the population as a whole? Not at all. First, they agreed to participate. They might have done so because they have a problem or fear that one exists. Also, the first 500 might be those who feel a sense of urgency, so they might represent the extreme cases. Although in some cases selecting people in this manner may produce a group that is *almost* representative, even the slightest bias will seriously impair the validity of your work and waste the effort invested in the study.

When sampling is properly done, each member of the population has an equal chance of being included in the study. The researcher samples the population; the members of the population may not modify the outcome of the sampling process once it is completed. If the subject of your investigation is skin allergies among children, for example, and you use a sampling technique, you cannot add or remove anyone, even if the two worst cases you know of were not selected in the sample. Further, only a breakdown in the sampling procedure that makes you suspect it was inappropriately done or biased would give you a reason to resample. This is an extremely rare problem, however, so you should not be critical of a sampling simply because certain individuals are not included.

You may have an intuitive problem with randomly sampling a population for a disease that we have already said does not occur randomly; however, the underlying factors contributing to adverse health effects will be randomly distributed in both the exposed and unexposed groups, so the nonrandomness of the disease process itself should not play a role in the distribution of the disease.

The Sampling Procedure
Sampling is done by obtaining a list of the members of the population and then randomly picking those to be surveyed. Each person

has an equal chance of being picked and, once chosen, must be included in the study. The first step of this process is often the most difficult: obtaining a complete list, a roster, of the population you have defined.

A roster of 2,000 names, as in our example, may be almost impossible to obtain. If you were investigating problems related to occupation, local unions might be able to provide membership lists; for elementary school children, school registration lists might be available through the schools or school board. There is no guarantee that these lists are absolutely correct, but they may be accurate enough that they will not introduce significant bias to the study. Two keys to building a roster are the type of list you are putting together and your ingenuity in obtaining material for it. (Some additional techniques will be introduced later about how to use other sources of materials.)

One technique that will greatly ease your work is to modify your roster—to convert your population into another unit of measure. Instead of a head count of individuals, you might consider listing households. Instead of defining your population as all individuals living within two miles of a chemical plant, you would then define it as all households within two miles of that plant, and you would thus reduce your roster to both a more manageable number and a more obtainable unit. (Street addresses are easier to obtain than names of all individuals in the community.) You can still ask questions about the individuals in the households and look at confounding factors and correlations within each household (age, sex, smoking, etc.), and you can still stratify according to exposure levels, but you will be considering exposure to the household. A roster of the population is easier to obtain in this manner, and the individuals in it can be approached in a more manageable way, yet the wide spectrum of individual differences that are characteristic of any community will still be taken into consideration.

As we stated at the beginning of this section, sampling of your roster (people, households, residential phone numbers, or whatever your population unit may be) is done randomly—you must choose some of these units to represent your population as a whole. A simple random sample is much like drawing names out of a hat, but with a large roster that becomes impractical. Random sampling can also be done by various other devices. They may sometimes look like a game, but they serve the purpose of achieving an unbiased selection of units from the population as a whole.

Random Number Table

Selecting units by means of a random number table is a paper-and-pencil method that achieves the same result as picking names out of a hat. It is done by applying numbers to a list arranged in an arbitrary but orderly manner—here, alphabetically. (The list in the example consists of individuals, but the technique is equally applicable to other population units.)

The following list is from our hypothetical population of 2,000.

1.	Abbott, L.	2.	Adams, M.
3.	Allison, G.	4.	Anderson, G.
5.	Atkins, B.	6.	Baker, S.
7.	Barnett, J.	8.	Benson, L.
9.	Brandt, W.	10.	Brown, G.
11.	Butler, H.	12.	Campbell, S.
13.	Cash, J.	14.	Clark, R.
15.	Coleman, R.	16.	Cortez, H.
17.	Cunningham, W.	18.	Daniels, H.
19.	Davis, M. . . .	2,000.	Zunick, B.

We can allow a random number table to dictate which names to choose. A random number table is simply a list of numbers, 00 to 99, arranged in columns and rows in random order. You could prepare your own random number table, but we have prepared one that you can apply in your study (table 4.1).

Sequential Sampling

Sequential sampling can be done by selecting from a roster at arbitrary intervals. A procedure as simple as taking every fourth unit could give you your sample of 500 from a population of 2,000. This is an easy method, and with a list of individuals, it is probably as random a sampling as you will ever need. If you were dealing with something like home addresses, however, this might not be satisfactory. Sequential sampling of a list of households by street and house number might produce a sample that included only houses on the same side of the street because of an odd/even street numbering system. This may not affect your study, but if the study is around a chemical dump, for example, excluding one side of the street may introduce bias.

Other Techniques

Dice rolls and coin flips are both simple examples of random processes that can easily be used in sampling. If you wanted your

Table 4.1   Use of a Table of Random Numbers

Problem / Procedure										
Problem Given a population of ninety cases, to select a random sample of twenty cases.	25	19	64	82	84	62	74	29	92	24
	23	02	41	46	04	44	31	52	43	07
	55	85	66	96	28	28	30	62	58	83
	68	45	19	69	59	35	14	82	56	80
	69	31	46	29	85	18	88	26	95	54
Procedure 1. Arbitrarily assign each case a number from 01 to 90.	37	31	62	28	98	94	61	47	03	10
	66	42	19	24	94	13	13	38	69	96
2. On the table of random numbers, arbitrarily pick a two-digit column.	33	65	78	12	35	91	59	11	38	44
	76	32	06	19	35	22	95	30	19	29
	43	33	42	02	59	20	39	84	95	61
3. With closed eyes, select a random start in that column.	28	31	93	43	94	87	73	19	38	47
	97	19	21	63	34	69	33	17	03	02
4. Beginning with the starting number, continue to sequentially select every two-digit number in that column (and in the next two-digit column, if necessary) until twenty cases have been selected.	82	80	37	14	20	56	39	59	89	63
	03	68	03	13	60	64	13	09	37	11
	65	16	58	11	01	98	78	80	63	23
	24	65	58	57	04	18	62	85	28	24
	02	72	64	07	75	85	66	48	38	73
	79	16	78	63	99	43	61	00	66	42
	04	75	14	93	39	68	52	16	83	34
5. In the event a random number not included in the sequence 01 to 90 occurs (e.g., 98), skip that number and proceed to the next random number listed.	40	64	64	57	60	97	00	12	91	33
	06	27	07	34	26	01	52	48	69	57
	62	40	03	87	10	96	88	22	46	04
	00	98	48	18	97	91	51	63	27	00
6. Similarly, if a random number already used occurs again, disregard it and continue to the next random number listed.	50	64	19	18	91	98	55	83	46	09
	38	54	52	25	78	01	98	00	89	85
	46	86	80	97	78	65	12	64	64	70
	90	72	92	93	10	09	12	81	93	00
7. To assure that a number is not picked twice, keep some record in numerical sequence of numbers selected.	66	21	41	77	60	99	35	72	61	22
	87	05	46	52	76	89	96	34	22	37
	46	90	61	03	06	89	85	33	22	80
	11	88	53	06	09	81	83	33	98	29
	11	05	92	06	97	68	82	34	08	83
	33	94	24	20	28	62	42	07	12	63
	24	89	74	75	61	61	02	73	36	85
	15	19	74	67	23	61	38	93	73	68
	05	64	12	70	88	80	58	35	06	88
	57	49	36	44	06	74	93	55	39	26
	77	82	96	96	97	60	42	17	18	48
	24	10	70	06	61	59	62	37	95	42
	50	00	07	78	23	49	54	36	85	14

Source: Anita K. Bahn, *Basic Medical Statistics* (Orlando, Fla.: Grune and Stratton, 1972). Used by permission of the publisher.

sample to include about one out of six people, you would simply roll one of the dice for each name on the list and then include only the names for which you rolled sixes.

One final sampling technique that may be of use is cluster sampling. A cluster sample assumes that the population is generally homogeneous and that any group of people or households you select will be representative of the population as a whole. So, instead of selecting individuals one by one, you choose small groups, or clusters. If your population is based on households, for example, you could use city blocks as the basis of your sampling. Surveying all the people on any one block is much easier than tracking down the same number of individual residences scattered throughout town. The key to using this method, however, is that the population must look very much the same over all, so that selecting one block over another does not influence the outcome of the survey. If major differences in social or socioeconomic character are found in the area, then cluster sampling is not appropriate.

If these techniques are ranked by effectiveness, a random number table is best if it is available. Other than that, a sequential technique is good if there is no reason it should be biased. Finally, a simple process such as rolling dice or flipping coins can be used to select people randomly for your study. Cluster sampling should be reserved for very homogeneous populations. If such a situation exists, then cluster sampling is a powerful and effective tool.

Sample Size

Since sampling is used when you are trying to reduce your work yet still arrive at some answers, you must decide how much work you can perform adequately (or wish to) and how difficult it will be to prove that a problem exists. As a guideline, if you can mobilize enough people to survey the entire population in a reasonable amount of time (say three months, though the time involved is really your decision), then try to do so. Nothing is as convincing as results based upon a survey of the entire population. You should not settle for surveying fewer than 200 people unless your entire population is smaller (as in small communities, occupationally related exposure, and other situations of confined exposure or effects).

The sample size will be a function of the type of information you are collecting. The rarer the disease or the more subtle the effect, the more people you will need to survey to demonstrate the presence of a health problem. If you are looking for an increase in skin allergies, for example (normally 10 percent of the population might be affected), and this increase seems to be a major one (three to five times greater than normal), then the 200 people suggested earlier should be sufficient to show that a problem does exist. If you were trying to demonstrate a doubling in the rate of brain tumors, however, you might have to survey a population of 10,000 to 15,000. Chapter 7, on data analysis, will explain the requirements for population size more fully and will help you determine how large a sample you need to have a reasonable chance of proving an effect. You must realize that some of these adverse health effects are going to be difficult to demonstrate, and so the more people you can possibly study the better.

Standards of Comparison

Selecting and surveying a population is not, alone, enough to prove that a community health hazard exists. You will need a standard of comparison, some measure of what is normal, against which to compare your findings. If you determine that the rate of cancer in your community is 34 percent this finding by itself does not permit you to draw any inference. But if you determine that it would be expected to be 25 percent on the basis of some known standard (or one you have developed), then the inference of an increased risk of cancer in your community is supportable. Three basic types of standards may be used: official health statistics, an actual comparison group of people, or the stratification technique mentioned earlier.

Health Statistics

The easiest way to gather baseline health data is from government statistics. All levels of government collect health data, which then are available to the public. The data are usually well analyzed for major causes of death or illness and are characterized with regard to contributing factors. Four main pitfalls may affect your use of health statistics: they may be taken from a population (state, county, etc.) that is entirely different in makeup from the population you are studying; the data may be significantly out of date; factors you might wish to take into account (such as age, sex, pregnancy) may not be reflected; and rarer types of disease or illness factors may not be listed or may be inadequately reported, which makes the health statistics useless to you.

Comparison Populations

Another baseline can be set up by putting together a comparison population (control group), a group of people that resembles your population in every way except for the factor you suspect represents an environmental hazard. This comparison population should have the same age and sex distribution and socioeconomic makeup as your study population; jobs should reflect the same types of work environments, and the social structure should be closely similar. What you hope to find is what the health status of your study population "should be." Any discrepancy between that and what you have observed may indicate an adverse environmental influence. Such a group may be hard to find and difficult to survey, but the strength a comparison population adds to your study is tremendous.

Stratification

Stratification separates your population into subsections arranged according to decreasing levels of exposure to the suspected pollutant. The group with the lowest level of exposure can serve to represent the normal background levels of certain disease states. It is not uncommon for such a subsection to be the most appropriate group obtainable for comparison as well as the one most easily defined.

Certain factors must be considered, however, when you plan to use stratification to obtain your baseline population: stratification assumes that the exposure source identified is actually the one at fault; good stratification implies that you have a clear grasp of what type of exposure is affecting the population and that you know the health effect of interest is significantly influenced by exposure to it. And proper stratification means that only the one pollutant is being considered and that no other pollutant is accidentally affecting the stratification.

The key to using stratification as your comparison technique is guessing right (by educated guesses or otherwise). If no differences can be found between the groups that are related to stratum (that is, level of exposure), you will have to seek other methods of comparison. Stratification is generally used to reinforce your suspicions about the exposure source (the closer the source, the worse the health effects). A second comparison technique (such as health statistics) should then be used on the study population as a whole.

A Hypothetical Study

The following scenario demonstrates some ways you can approach a problem.

Our hypothetical couple, the Wilsons, live in the town of Jackson. Their second child has recently been in the hospital for minor problems associated with neurological disorders: occasional dizziness, nausea, blurred vision, and so on—just six weeks after a sibling was similarly affected. A casual remark by the clinic nurse that "something must be going around" caught Mrs. Wilson's attention. Though their first child had complained of similar problems, no medical problem had been identified, and the symptoms continued to follow a pattern of recurrence and resolution over the subsequent weeks. Mrs. Wilson observed that bed rest seemed to eliminate the problems but that when the child was up and about, visiting friends and playing outdoors, the symptoms returned. The child also had apparently become aware of this, because for the past week or more he had chosen to remain indoors, content to play with toys and ask friends to come over.

Mrs. Wilson then made inquiries among friends, and uncovered two similar accounts from parents in the same neighborhood as well as an observation that some elderly people had recently begun to develop respiratory problems. Over the next two weeks the series of stories began to infuse Mrs. Wilson with a sense of urgency, since the more she learned the more she was convinced that the poor health of her community was excessive.

Jackson is a community of 38,000 that has two major chemical production plants as well as seven or eight smaller chemical production units. The great majority of local employment is in some aspect of these chemical industries, and the overall socioeconomic pattern of the community is fairly uniform except for one region where the employees of higher rank live (manager, unit supervisor, and so on). The plants themselves are clustered along the river and form a fairly consolidated industrial complex.

The more Mrs. Wilson thought about the community health problems, the more she came to believe they were associated in some way with the chemical plants, though she had no way of knowing which plant was responsible. When she shared her concerns with other residents, however, she met a fair amount of cynicism, though she was able to recruit a few concerned individuals. The Jackson Citizens for Community Health, as Mrs. Wilson's group called themselves, was formed and began studying the health status of the residents of Jackson. This is how the group approached the task.

Step 1. Defining the Problems

Problem 1.   To determine if the health status of the Jackson community is poorer than it should be.

Problem 2.   If the health status is indeed poorer, to determine whether this effect is associated with the chemical plants in the area.

Step 2. Developing an Approach

One option was to try to draw attention to their suspicions through the local and regional media. This method is usually ineffective, however, and tends not to solve anything. The other choice was to try to demonstrate that the health problem was real and that the chemical plants might have something to do with it. Though public services might assist in many cases, as they did with Mrs. Wilson, community members must start the process themselves.

Step 3. Generating a Health Survey

With the help of various resource materials and individual input, a study to survey the community's health was pieced together.

Step 4. Formulating a Hypothesis

Mrs. Wilson's group formulated a hypothesis:

1. The community suffers adverse health conditions at a higher rate than expected.
2. These adverse health conditions are directly related to chemical exposure from the chemical plants in the industrial complex.
3. The frequency of adverse effects in various measures of health is directly related to proximity of residences to the chemical plants.

Mrs. Wilson's group has ruled out occupation as a possible source of chemical exposure because it was not immediately obvious. They took advantage of a concept of dosage, however, by proposing that the effect was related to proximity to the chemical plants. They also proposed that the community of Jackson was different, in general, from normal communities so that the lack of a demonstrable adverse effect from the chemical plants would not nullify the possibility that Jackson might have a serious health problem.

Step 5. Defining the Population

The first step Mrs. Wilson took was to define the population as all residents of the town of Jackson (excluding the upper-middle-class to upper-class area at the east edge of town). Patterns of illness can sometimes follow socioeconomic patterns, and for the sake of homogeneity in the study population this small sector of the community was excluded. Impoverished neighborhoods were also excluded because they pose a similar problem. This is not to say that these groups did not have health problems or that the citizens' group was not concerned about these areas. It was simply that in Jackson most people were of the same basic socioeconomic group, and concentrating on a large, homogeneous population would result in an easier, more significant study. Concentrating on small, unique groups may be more difficult because of confounding factors, and a comparison population is not easy to obtain. If the study population is shown to have an abnormal health status, however, concern should be voiced for the health status of the other two groups.

Using the individual as the basis of the population causes various problems: in generating a roster, if one chooses to sample; in locating subjects, if one chooses to stratify the population; and in obtaining responses, if minors or infants are part of the population. As a consequence, Mrs. Wilson's group chose to define the population by households, keeping the same constraints as before. Using a detailed city map, they identified the areas in Jackson that were to be used as the basis of the population. According to available census data, these areas now encompassed 32,000 people in about 9,000 households.

Step 6. Stratifying the Population

Because Mrs. Wilson believed the health problems were associated in some way with the chemical plants, she decided to divide the population into three groups based on how close they lived to the chemical complex: within a mile and a half of the plants; between a mile and a half and three miles of the plants; and three miles or more away. These were called zones 1, 2, and 3. Zone 1 contained 2,880 people in 810 households; zone 2 had 6,400 people in 1,800 households; and zone 3 had 22,720 people in 6,390 households.

Step 7. Defining the Control Population

The Built-in Control Group

If an adverse health effect indeed proves to be related to living near the chemical plants, then the stratification process described in step 6 will result in a built-in control group and will also indicate that the chemical plants are at fault.

The Outside Comparison Group
Since the health effects observed up to this point could indicate
a number of illnesses, compiled health statistics could not readily
be used as a basis of comparison. What Mrs. Wilson did was to
identify another community, Franklin—eight miles from Jackson
and with 18,000 people—that was of essentially the same socioeconomic level but whose economy was based on a heavy machine
assembly plant. She applied the same selection criteria to this
group that she used in Jackson and came up with about 4,200
households that could serve as an appropriate comparison group
for her study.

Step 8. Sample Size
The general rule of at least 200 households per study group is probably a good starting point for sample size. Mrs. Wilson needed to
sample approximately 200 households from each stratum as well
as at least 200 households from the comparison group in Franklin.
Because the comparison group is so important in establishing the
baseline health status, the statistics generated for it need to be
even more precise than those for the study population. Mrs. Wilson finally decided to sample 200 households in each of zones 1
and 2 in Jackson and 300 households each in zone 3 and in the
comparison population of Franklin.

Step 9. Sampling Technique
Using detailed city maps of both towns, Mrs. Wilson established
residential blocks either by using streets or by introducing arti-
ficial boundaries where courts or circles disturbed the traditional
concept of a residential block. Once all the blocks were identified, they were labeled and rosters were generated for each zone
and for the town of Franklin as well. A block averaged twelve
households. Using cluster sampling, seventeen blocks were randomly chosen out of each of zones 1 and 2, and twenty-five blocks
were selected from zone 3 and from Franklin. These households
constituted the people who would be surveyed.

Since Mrs. Wilson occasionally found that one of the blocks
sampled turned out to be commercial, she specified that when a
block proved to have more than 25 percent business enterprises or
fewer than six homes it would be excluded and a new block
selected.

Step 10. Surveying the Population

This step will be covered in succeeding chapters. Once you have reached this point, you have completed the major part of the study design. During analysis, you can concentrate on specific subpopulations that you find of interest.

One problem you may encounter is how to motivate the comparison population to participate in the study. You could do this by emphasizing how the study might benefit them by revealing health problems that might be beginning in their neighborhoods. We will address the question of promoting subject participation later.

You may also find that the comparison population is a good distance away and requires a large amount of work to survey. Planning and organization can make this process easier to execute. As we mentioned before, although comparison populations are difficult to deal with, they are definitely the most desirable way to establish baseline health statistics.

5   What Information Do You Need?
Questionnaire Design, Administration, and Limitations

Barbara L. Harper
Mary C. Lowery

he purpose of the health survey is twofold: to let you conclude with some degree of certainty that a health problem does or does not exist in your community and, if it appears that one does exist, to provide enough information to convince state or federal officials that this is true. You will first need historical, physical, and demographic (characteristics describing the residents) information. You will also need to approach resource individuals and groups. The conduct of the survey itself will depend on the preliminary information you collect, how much you know about the suspected problem, and the number of volunteers available to administer the survey. As a first step, a series of nonrandom interviews of some of the most severely affected people, using your entire questionnaire, will tell you many things: how many people are being affected, what the most prevalent symptoms are and how severely and frequently they occur, and so on. Since the questionnaire we provide (chap. 6) was designed to be applicable to diverse situations, certain questions may not be needed in particular cases, and certain sections (occupational, for instance) are not applicable to certain individuals (nonworking mothers and children). However, it is usually better to have too much information than too little, so proceed cautiously if you decide to shorten

84

the questionnaire. For a community-organized health survey, it will probably be most convenient to make contact with the households to be surveyed, deliver the questionnaire in person, let the members of the household fill it in at their convenience, then retrieve the questionnaire in person and answer any questions that have arisen. You must consider how you can ensure that individual answers will be kept confidential, while still being able to pinpoint symptoms on a map. You must also be aware of the limitations of any kind of health survey. First, the people who do not return the questionnaire are not a representative sample of your community. Second, knowing that your community may be exposed to something often leads to a more careful survey than is done in the unexposed group. Third, the conditions reported in the survey will probably not be verified by physician or hospital records, so you will be relying on lay individuals to report symptoms and on other lay individuals to code the answers. Finally, as you collect information, certain questions will be raised and inferences made that you will have to answer. These largely arise from the attempt to extrapolate the results you obtain for your entire community (probably expressed as an *average* for the neighborhood or community) to individual cases. Since there are certain natural background rates for each condition, you will not be able to say with 100 percent certainty that a particular case was directly caused by chemical X. By preparing your answers to these kinds of questions, you should be able to alleviate some of the trauma that inevitably arises when you conclude that an adverse environmental health effect exists.

This chapter will acquaint you with methods for collecting needed information, both health related and community related. The next chapter includes a questionnaire that can be used as a preliminary health survey and that, if necessary, can be shortened for a larger survey once you are sure which medical conditions are most prevalent in your community. Specific instructions for administering the questionnaire are given, and limitations of health surveys are discussed. Remember, your purpose in conducting this survey will be to document the incidence of some of the most prevalent conditions of concern in your community, not the exact incidence of every symptom. A high-quality, well-documented survey that indicates a significant increase in a few key conditions should be enough to convince state officials to conduct a full-scale investigation to pinpoint the chemical culprit. On the other hand, a high-quality well-documented survey that indicates there is *not* a significant increase in the key conditions should relieve doubts and tension within the community. Whatever the outcome, your group owes it to itself and to the community to do a good job, and we firmly believe this is within the capability of intelligent citizens.

At this point you will have formed a community organization and begun to focus on specific issues. Before actually beginning to collect your data, however, some preliminary research is in order, if you have not already done this. Take advantage of city services to collect information on whichever of the following items are pertinent to your situation.

The Chamber of Commerce and other offices in city hall can provide information on the economic and tax bases of your town and on the major employers, and they should be able to give you a breakdown of employers by type of industry and tell you whether they have filed permits to emit or discharge waste and so on. The archives of your library can supply old city directories and other material on local history—this will tell you what industries existed in the past (and where), the approximate age of housing (when water lines were put in), and similar items. A detailed city map combined with census tract figures (obtainable in the reference section of your local library) will help you define your population sample groups and may suggest additional factors to consider in your survey. Also match the map to terrain: elevation, drainage patterns, wind patterns, vegetation, and natural and man-made bodies of water. Note land-use patterns (farming, mining) and compare them with earlier patterns (for example, an earlier industrial site may now be residential, a land fill may be a school playground). Your library will have a wealth of information of this sort and can guide you to local historical groups or knowledgeable individuals who may prove to be valuable resources and save you a lot of time. City (and state) planners will also have similar information used for forecasting, but they may not be enthusiastic about sharing it if it appears to them that you are trying to prove it is hazardous to live in their town. Use common sense and remain carefully neutral and objective when asking for help from someone who might have something to lose, tangible or otherwise.

Another resource you may approach with more or less success is local health professionals (family physicians, pediatricians, general practitioners, paramedics), who may have already noticed something and may even discuss particular symptoms you should include in the questionnaire. Local health officials may also be willing to help. Not only is it common courtesy to advise these groups in advance that you will be conducting an environmental health survey, but it will also increase the likelihood of their later support and cooperation should you find that a problem exists. These groups tend to be cautious and conservative, but they should react favorably to an objective, high-quality survey even if it is conducted by a nonmedical group.

During these initial stages you will begin focusing on just what questions you hope to answer. Two general situations might arise: (1) you know there is a (potential) source of pollution but don't know if it has caused any adverse health effects; (2) you suspect too high an incidence of illness but don't know if it is real or don't know of any reason for it. Often the actual situation is a combination of the two: you think there is a problem and have already assigned the blame to a particular source (a trap you should be careful to avoid in the interest of objectivity, especially since your assumptions may eventually be disproved).

The actual conduct of the survey, and your sample sizes in particular, will depend on your particular situation. We cannot hope to address every possibility that may arise, but we will give examples and guidelines so that you should be able to proceed without difficulty. A number of community situations are possible:

1. You are absolutely sure you have collected every case of a major or a usually rare disease in your community (such as childhood leukemia) and know your total population size and age distribution. In this case you can quickly calculate an incidence rate, as described in chapter 7.

2. Your community or division numbers fewer than 250 households, and you have enough volunteers to survey every household. You will need to find a comparable control (unexposed) group, as described in the previous chapter.

3. Your community is too large for you to survey everyone, but you suspect that everyone is equally exposed. You will need to survey a cross section by random selection to be sure that the incidence of disease accurately represents the incidence in the community as a whole.

4. Your community is not evenly exposed: (a) You have a point source of pollution, and the farther away the residence, the less exposure there is. The previous chapter described how to "stratify,"

or assess the effect of distance from the source on incidence of health problems. (*b*) You have a point source of pollution with unequal exposures in different directions, usually characteristic of air pollution or pollution of a river or stream. In this case you will have to "stratify" differently in different directions (upwind or downwind, or by quadrant).

5. You do not know how the community is exposed, or whether health effects, if any, are evenly distributed, or whether the pollution occurs evenly or unevenly. Pinpointing cases on a map will be one of your tools in this case.

At this point you will probably want to conduct a small series of "open" or "unfocused" interviews. This "discovery" procedure will alert you to particular facets of your situation (symptoms, environmental clues, the history and scope of the problem, etc.). A medically skilled interviewer is beneficial here to relate symptoms to organ systems and exposures, and also because open interviews like this depend on recall. You will be collecting a lot of hearsay anecdotes, which do have limited use as an overview even though they are not scientific or admissible in court. If you have no one skilled in any sort of interviewing, your task force or steering committee will need to use the entire questionnaire as is, and you will probably want to do some background reading from the various references in this manual. If you need to use a large sample and are short on volunteers, you may wish to consider using this questionnaire as a preliminary survey of twenty-five or so most affected people to collect all symptoms that are appearing. From this you can formulate a short version concentrating primarily on a few key conditions. Don't be in too great a hurry to eliminate seemingly irrelevant questions, however, since a chemical can affect different people in different ways. A complete preliminary survey should nevertheless be sufficient to uncover the most common symptoms (which will be enough for you to prove your point). If you are sure that you are concerned only with one or a few specific conditions, you may even condense the questionnaire into a page or two, short enough to fill out by telephone, as described later. Use your common sense in choosing what questions to ask: an air pollution route of exposure means you may find respiratory symptoms and certain environmental clues that you would not find in waterborne exposures, while waterborne contaminants may lead to intestinal symptoms and fish kills. Again, however, just because you know of the presence of one airborne chemical you must not assume that that chemical is necessarily the only cause of the problems; they may actually be caused in part by another entirely unrelated waterborne chemical, for example.

Questionnaire Design

We have compiled our questionnaire using material from a number of large, well-tested questionnaires and have added some environmental questions. That most of the questions have been field tested means we will not have to summarize the entire area of questionnaire design, itself the subject of many professional books. Some of these texts are listed in the References for those who wish further information.

We have tried to design the questionnaire to be as widely applicable as possible, and therefore we have had to make some assumptions both about the exposed group and about what kind of data you will want to collect. First, both acute and chronic conditions are included; this concept is very important with respect to the end points you are measuring. Symptoms of chronic exposure may resemble, in a milder form, symptoms of acute poisoning by the same agent. Some symptoms may be slowly progressive so that their onset cannot be pinpointed. Adverse birth outcomes obviously have more or less a nine-month waiting period. Cancer, however, has a variable latency, with few or no symptoms appearing in the interim. Since it may take five to forty years for some cancers to develop, there are many problems in obtaining estimates of exposures that occurred far in the past. Occupational histories should therefore extend back as far as possible; we have allowed space for a complete occupational history since age sixteen plus detailed questions for more acute (past five years) exposures.

Finally, the length of the questionnaire is less important than question content; though it may seem long, you still have the option of adding questions based on your own open interviews.

Administration

The major question to be decided at this point is whether the questionnaire will be administered by an interviewer or will be self-administered. Several studies comparing the two have found that self-administered questionnaires are generally just as valid, and a little more valid on sensitive questions (Siemiatycki 1979). Optimal response will probably be generated by making initial contact by mail or telephone, then mailing (or hand delivering) the questionnaire and using an interviewer only for persistent non-responders. You may be criticized for not using an interviewer for every questionnaire or for using several different interviewers (if your sample size is small enough to allow you to interview everyone). Probably the major problem of your entire project will be how to ensure high-quality data when laypeople report their symptoms to nonmedical interviewers or scorers. Untrained interviewers may also be biased, especially in a local setting where they know about exposures and what symptoms might be expected. For those reasons, unless you are overwhelmed with skilled volunteer interviewers, the questionnaire should probably be self-administered. The questionnaire can thus be filled in at the convenience of the household, will not need to be completed in one sitting, and will allow respondents time to look up personal medical records. You may choose to limit contact to the initial telephone call and have subjects mail the questionnaires back in, or you may prefer to pick up the questionnaires and at the same time answer any questions there might be. Even better, you may hand deliver the questionnaires and review them with the respondents, who will then fill in the appropriate sections at their convenience.

The first step in the health survey itself will be to verify addresses and send a "preletter." The letter should look as professional as possible, depending on funds. Perhaps a printing business would donate paper and print a letterhead, the letter itself, or the questionnaire; if any businesses or groups have agreed to be sponsors, include them somewhere in the letterhead. The preletter not only is a courtesy, it increases the response rate. This letter will describe the group and its history, tell subjects they will be receiving the questionnaire, explain its purpose, and tell why your group is conducting the survey, why people should participate, how they were chosen and of which groups they are members, how individual responses will be kept confidential, how the results will be used, and whether respondents can expect any benefits. Offer to send a summary report (at the end of the questionnaire you may ask whether respondents would like a summary of the results).

A short time after the initial letter is sent, you may want to telephone each household to ask if the letter has arrived, explain how important it is that they participate, and ask if they are willing. Have a phone number and references ready.

At this point you will already realize that nonparticipants are proving to be a problem. Every epidemiologic study is plagued with nonparticipants. They present a particular difficulty when they are part of a random sample that must accurately represent your entire community. Strictly speaking, once subjects have been chosen as part of a random sample, they must remain part of that sample. The nonparticipant should not be replaced by another randomly selected person. The reason for this derives from the reasons people do not want to participate: they do not have a problem, they do not perceive that anyone else has a real problem, they have a health problem but do not want to admit it, they perceive the survey as an attack on their employer and therefore on their job security, and so on. In other words, the nonparticipants may have a different makeup than the rest of your community, and their nonparticipation may cause inaccuracies in your calculations. By repeatedly approaching these people as your study progresses, perhaps you will succeed in convincing them to participate. The few who absolutely refuse may at that point be replaced from your list of alternates, also chosen randomly. Remember, however, that if you are concerned about a sensitive condition (sterility, for example), your nonparticipants may include proportionally more affected people than you would expect based on the rate you establish for the rest of the community. Another important point: if your random selection includes people who have recently moved away because of health effects and you cannot reach them, you may miss some of the most severely affected cases.

You are now ready to deliver the questionnaire. Attached to the front of each questionnaire will be a cover letter, which should be neat, official-looking, short, and to the point. It will review the nature of the study and tell how the data will be used, and it will include particular instructions. Ask that it be returned as soon as possible rather than by a firm deadline; this will avoid having people think it is too late to turn it in at all. If the questionnaire is delivered and returned by mail, enclose an addressed return envelope (stamped, not metered). An actual sample cover letter is not supplied with the questionnaire because details will vary with each survey. General instructions are supplied at the front of the questionnaire.

There are two additional points to consider before the questionnaires are sent. First is the possibility of including an unannounced "incentive" with the questionnaire, which creates a sense of obligation to fill it out. If your funds will not permit enclosing money, perhaps businesses will donate discount coupons, certificates for free hamburgers, or something else people are likely to appreciate.

The second point that will need careful consideration is the issue of confidentiality and anonymity. True anonymity (in which case you really do not know who has answered and who has not) will probably not be applicable to most environmental situations, though large random-sample surveys usually adhere to it. You will need to know the exact or approximate address of each household (at least which block and perhaps which side of the block) so that residence and symptoms can be correlated. There are a number of ways to handle this. First, you can ask for name and address and assure the people of confidentiality. Second, you can assign each household a number (being careful that the right code number goes into each envelope) and keep the code numbers and matched names and addresses in a locked safe, safe-deposit box, or other secure place. Third, you can keep names and addresses separate so that you can map symptoms without connecting them to names and faces.

Three to five days after mailing the questionnaire, mail postcards thanking subjects for participating (and reminding them to fill them in if they have not). Obviously you will have to know who has returned the questionnaire and who hasn't in order to follow up nonrespondents. At this point don't be afraid to be persistent (but not obnoxious), since these reminders are a very effective technique for improving response rate. Let nonrespondents know that their response is really needed. You may need to hand deliver another questionnaire or have an interviewer administer it. Follow-ups may be humorous postcards or telephone calls. Remember, these are your data and it is important to your efforts and those of numerous volunteers.

Limitations

Let us briefly discuss some of the drawbacks pertaining to the quality of data obtained by using this particular questionnaire. The first major criticism you may encounter will be for the lack of interviewers (if you have not used interviewers at all) or for using untrained or semitrained interviewers (if you have). As we discussed above, the only way to counter this objection with limited local resources is to make every effort to remain nonbiased, to avoid asking leading questions or digging for symptoms just because you know a person has been exposed, and to write down everything you plan to say ahead of time so it will always be the same. This weakness will remain a point of contention, but with common sense and close supervision it can be minimized.

The second weakness will be lack of verification by a physician of either symptoms or conditions. The survey information will be collected from laypeople by other laypeople, and furthermore it relies largely on recall. Accuracy is proportional to overall self-awareness of current symptoms and also to people's ability to remember names of major diseases. Whether a medical interviewer would improve data quality or not, however, is in doubt: medical doctors classify fewer patients as having priority health problems than do the patients themselves (Bennett and Richie 1975), and local doctors are often not the ones who first recognize a general health problem.

Other limitations are inherent in any questionnaire. Reasons for not responding to a questionnaire include language barriers, migrancy, and racial, cultural, and literacy factors. On the other hand, a person may have good health and not perceive a problem or any need to determine if there is a problem for others. Bad health may physically interfere with answering. Those who do not bother to take care of their general health may not want to answer a health-related questionnaire. People also tend to report better or more socially desirable habits than they have, so recreational drug use, smoking, drinking, and so on will be underreported to some degree. Some types of questions, especially on reproduction, are usually answered less accurately, as are certain conditions that may still carry a social stigma. In occupational histories, lower job satisfaction is correlated with overreporting of symptoms. Length of residence itself is a variable in that affected persons move away first and less sensitive ones stay, and the same thing pertains to occupations (sensitive people self-select themselves out of uncomfortable jobs). People may also move out of the area at retirement or if they become disabled.

One final factor that will probably remain with you throughout your investigation is the bias introduced as soon as a person knows he may be exposed to something. He may find out through the local newspaper, from your initial contact, or from his neighbors. Your group should discuss this from the outset and agree on answers that will not cause undue alarm yet will be as accurate as possible. People in the control group will want to know if they are exposed (answer: not to the factors that you are studying, as far as you are aware). Exposed or potentially exposed people will want to know about the exposure (to what, how much, how often). You probably will not have had a water or air analysis done, but, if you have, can you reasonably withhold this from them? In terms of statistical validity, knowing which group they are in instantly biases people's answers. There is usually underreporting of symptoms in controls and overreporting in exposed subjects unless the condition is so clear-cut that this is not a factor (you either have cancer or you don't). When people know they have been exposed, poorer health is not only acceptable but almost expected. Known exposure can also be a built-in excuse for poor health or poor health habits. Questions are bound to arise during the course of your study, such as: Why are you asking about my hobbies? Did this cause my baby's birth defect? Did my husband bring home poisonous chemicals on his clothes? and so on. You will be asked how you can link one chemical to its particular *health* effects in individuals if you cannot say one way or another what caused a particular *birth* defect. The answer is a statistical one: the degree of increase of a particular condition that a certain exposure is "likely" to produce *in a population* is not really applicable to individual cases. Remember the analogy of contributory factors filling up a person's bottles until one overflows and a disease develops (chap. 2).

To give some perspective on this issue, we will use an imaginary example: suppose that in the air of a suburb of a large city a known animal carcinogen has been identified. Of the 20,000 people in that suburb, 18,000 "feel fine." (This is hypothetical, of course, since it is not practical to ascertain the health status of all 20,000 residents.) Of the 2,000 who feel less than fine, the symptoms of 1,950 can be attributed to "natural" causes (old age, infections, etc.) and occur with the same frequency as in the unexposed control group. Of the fifty whose health problems cannot be explained by any nonenvironmental cause, fifteen have intermittent skin rashes, fifteen have neurological symptoms, five have nonspecific lung problems, five have digestive problems, five have cancer of various sites, and five have serious chemical sensitivity or allergic reactions. The point here is that, even when contamination is verified, most people show neither acute nor chronic toxicity. How about permanent genetic effects? Let us suppose that instead of five expected cases of a particular kind of cancer, you find ten (statistical analysis will tell you if this is "real" or not); again, almost everyone does *not* now have cancer. How many people currently being exposed can be expected to develop this kind of cancer in the future as a result of being exposed now? Again, very few: perhaps twenty more instead of the ten more that would develop this kind of cancer anyway. Will these cases of cancer develop earlier than they otherwise would? Perhaps, but the multitude of factors contributing to the cancer process (chap. 2) makes this question impossible to answer with our current level of understanding. Suppose you uncover a slight excess of low birth weight and spontaneous abortion (miscarriage). The same answers can be used: most births are *not* affected, many factors contribute to the final outcome, and there is a certain "natural" incidence (i.e., we cannot yet explain the mechanism). Your community group must be prepared to explain these concepts to everyone involved, so that they do not think they are cancer time bombs or that they can avoid birth defects if they move away from the area. On the other hand, if your final report concludes that there is no evidence of an environmental health problem, you may have to explain why someone develops cancer anyway. Again, the purpose of the health survey is to determine if there is a statistically "real" problem so that health authorities can justify a complete survey.

Summary: Excess in a Few Key Conditions

The questionnaire we provide is somewhat limited in terms of assessing chronic diseases, including cancer. As we mentioned before, there are special considerations in regard to diseases that take a long time to develop. If an environmental survey eventually results in court action in an attempt to compensate the victims of chronic disease or to punish the toxic waste generator (see chap. 9), supplementary information will be necessary. For instance, a complete residential history for each victim would be taken, which would address questions of other exposures and how long a person must have lived in the community to be included as a party to the legal action (in a class action suit). On the other hand, a complete occupancy history for the community (from tax assessor roles) and extensive tracking of people who lived in the community during times of potential exposure will also probably be necessary. All these considerations pertain to determining possible causes of the condition whose current incidence rate you have already established.

Epidemiology is largely common sense. You know your community situation better than anyone else, so rely on your own judgment in choosing which health effects to concentrate on. Remember, all you need do is accurately measure a few of the most prevalent symptoms in the community, so focus on what you have discovered from your preliminary survey. Naturally, state health officials will have to spend more effort on a cancer cluster than on skin rashes; on the other hand, they may choose to spend their limited funds on a well-documented large increase in dermatitis rather than on an unsubstantiated cluster of birth defects.

No perfect epidemiologic study has ever been conducted, and probably none will be. But if you arm yourself with an objective, rational approach and know the advantages and limitations of your study design before you begin, there is no reason your study cannot be as good as most and better than many. Remember, you owe it to yourself and to your neighbors to conduct your study as professionally as possible, whether you use the entire questionnaire or condense it to a few pages. A well-conducted study should save you considerable time, expense, and emotional stress, whether you document the existence of a problem or eliminate unfounded fears. You can do it.

Part 2

The First Phase
Practical Guidelines for a
General Health Survey

6   **How to Get the Information**
The Questionnaire,
Question Discussion,
and Tabulation

Barbara L. Harper
Mary C. Lowery
Michael J. Scott
Paul Mills

his chapter is divided into two main sections: the questionnaire and a discussion of each question, and instructions on
coding the answers and transferring them to the tabulation forms.
The questionnaire itself is presented here in its complete form.
The discussion describes why each question was included, what
kind of information it asks for, and how important it is. If your
group does not have the resources to administer and tabulate the
entire questionnaire, certain questions can be answered in advance
or can be left out altogether if they clearly do not pertain to your
particular situation. Coding each answer to be entered on tabulation sheets is essential for reducing to one page the amount of
paperwork for each person in your sample. Each person (man,
woman, or child) will use one tabulation form, so that results can
be expressed individually. Thus results for a mother will include
some information on her children, but the children will be tabulated by themselves so that the general health questions in section A can be tabulated for the children as well as for the parents.
When you are finished, you should therefore have one tabulation
form *per person,* as discussed in the next chapter. Although this

chapter may look intimidating, if you proceed through each part in order, the entire procedure should become clear.

First, we need to reemphasize a few general items concerning this questionnaire. As we explained earlier, the medical terminology included in the questionnaire elicits the fact that a person knows he has a particular condition because a doctor has told him so. This is an indirect way of confirming diagnosis by a physician without access to physician or hospital records. Of course, responsible physicians may help families fill out the forms, but since this is often not possible, the questionnaire has been designed so as not to require a physician's assistance.

A second point to consider before beginning your survey is whether you are simply measuring adverse health effects or whether you want to examine as many variables as possible as a first step in searching for the causes of any such effects you find. Obviously, if you do not ask about occupation, you will not know if occupation contributes to adverse health effects. The questions you leave out now will have to be asked eventually, by you or by whatever agency comes to your assistance. Therefore, unless you are extremely short of manpower, we recommend asking as many questions as you can in a single sampling. You will not have to analyze all the results right away, since your primary goal is to determine whether there is an adverse health effect, but you will have the information you need when you want to look at other variables.

Last, this questionnaire is primarily designed to ask, Who has what now? In other words, it assesses acute or permanent effects. Chronic conditions such as cancer or other progressive diseases will be detected only in those who currently have them. One question asks about household members who have died in the past five years, but other than this there is no mechanism for measuring death rates from any cause. Finding out about former household members who died more than five years ago and knowing how long they lived in the community before death is a complex procedure. Even professional epidemiologists often cannot agree on how many people lived in one particular place, worked in another, were exposed to a certain amount of some chemical, and died of a particular cause. This process entails collecting complete residential, occupational, and exposure histories as well as making a rigorous examination of death certificates, and it is generally beyond the resources of community groups. The more information you can get on annual mortality rates in past years (city, county, or state records) the better, but if you cannot obtain them on your own, these answers will have to wait until the next phase (see chap. 8).

Environmental Health Questionnaire

This questionnaire is designed to assess the health status of individual households. It is divided into four sections:

  A. Family description and general health, filled in for each person
  B. Occupation and life-style, all adults
  C. Reproductive history, all adult women
  D. Children's health. Sections A and D should be filled in for children.

It may be administered by an interviewer or may be self-administered. The time for completion will vary from about thirty minutes (young, single, nonparent) upward.

College students may answer appropriate sections if they are now at home, especially if they recently lived in this household full time.

Section A: The important factor in this section is whether any conditions reported have been diagnosed by a doctor.

Section B: A complete occupational history for each person is followed by more detailed questions on jobs held during the past five years. If the person has never worked, skip the occupational part and proceed to the neighborhood description.

Section C: This section and the next concern only children who currently live with you. Each adult woman (over eighteen years old) who lives in the household should answer this section.

If there has never been a pregnancy, stop at question 11. If there has been a pregnancy, even if it did not end in birth, answer all the questions you can in this section, since many concern early pregnancy and the time before pregnancy.

Section D: Some of these questions will not apply to infants or very young children. Answer all you can for each child up to age eighteen.

Attach a continuation page at the end of the questionnaire if more space is needed for any question, or if you have any comments on your particular situation.

Thank you for your time and patience.

For more information, call _____

The Health Detective's Handbook: A Guide to the Investigation of Environmental Health Hazards by Nonprofessionals, edited by Marvin S. Legator, Barbara L. Harper, and Michael J. Scott. © 1985 The Johns Hopkins University Press. This questionnaire may be reproduced without permission.

Section A. Family Description and General Health

The first part of this section inquires about some variables known to be important for epidemiologic studies. The description of the family and family medical history may be filled in once per family, but questions A11 through A19 must be answered for each person. The family medical history is concerned with blood relatives, not step-relatives. A lengthy list of symptoms and diagnosed conditions must be filled out for each person. Since these conditions may not be verified from hospital, physician, or other records, the year of diagnosis *by a doctor* is important. A record of major medications is also important, since drugs have many side effects and can interact with each other.

Name
_____

Address
_____

Telephone
_____

or Identification number

A1. Race
- ☐ 1. White (not Hispanic)
- ☐ 2. Black
- ☐ 3. Hispanic
- ☐ 4. Native American
- ☐ 5. Oriental
- ☐ 6. Other

A2. Type of neighborhood
- ☐ 1. Urban
- ☐ 2. Suburban
- ☐ 3. Town or village
- ☐ 4. Mixed industrial/residential
- ☐ 5. Farm or rural

A3. Total household income
- ☐ 1. Below $10,000
- ☐ 2. $10,000–$20,000
- ☐ 3. $20,000–$30,000
- ☐ 4. $30,000–$50,000
- ☐ 5. Over $50,000

A4. Type of housing
- ☐ 1. Single-family
- ☐ 2. Multifamily
- ☐ 3. Mobile home

A5. What year did you move to your present address?_____

A6. What year did you move into this community?_____

A7. How many persons regularly live in your household?_____

A8. Has anyone (within the last five years) left this household owing to death?
Who? Cause of death?

_____

_____

A9. For other reasons? Who? Reason for leaving?

_____

_____

A10. Source of water
   ☐ 1. City   ☐ 3. Bottled
   ☐ 2. Well   ☐ 4. Unknown

A11. Age _____

A12. Sex
   ☐ Male
   ☐ Female

A13. Height in inches _____

A14. Weight in pounds _____

A15. Last grade of school completed_____

A16. Did you serve in the armed forces?
   ☐ 1. Army   ☐ 4. Marines
   ☐ 2. Navy   ☐ 5. Other
   ☐ 3. Air Force

A17. Year entered service (do not count Reserves)_____

A18. Year left active service_____

    or still in service _____

A19. Longest tour of duty
   ☐ 1. Europe   ☐ 4. Africa
   ☐ 2. North America   ☐ 5. Asia
   ☐ 3. South America   ☐ 6. Other

A20. Family medical history (place checks where appropriate)

	Male parent or respondent	Your father	Your mother	Your brother	Your brother	Your sister	Your sister	Any first cousins	Your grandparents	Other	Female parent or respondent	Your father	Your mother	Your brother	Your brother	Your sister	Your sister	Any first cousins	Your grandparents	Other	
a																					Allergies
b																					Anemia
c																					Arthritis/gout
d																					Asthma
e																					Bleeding/bruising
f																					Cancer or tumors
g																					Convulsions/epilepsy
h																					Diabetes
i																					Drinking or drug problem
j																					Eczema
k																					Emphysema
l																					Heart trouble
m																					Hepatitis
n																					High blood pressure
o																					Frequent infections
p																					Kidney or bladder problems
q																					Mental illness
r																					Migraines
s																					Abnormal menstrual periods
t																					Psoriasis
u																					Pneumonia
v																					Polio
w																					Prostate problems
x																					Rheumatic fever
y																					Stomach or intestinal disease
z																					Stroke
aa																					Thyroid problems
bb																					Tuberculosis
cc																					Ulcers
dd																					Veneral disease
ee																					Weight problem

1 2 3 4 5 6 7 8 9 10 11 12 13 14 15 16 17 18

A21. Lung
Diagnosed conditions
Year of occurrence or diagnosis

_____ 1. Tuberculosis

_____ 2. Persistent bronchitis

_____ 3. Pneumoconiosis

_____ 4. Lung disease

_____ 5. Pneumonia

_____ 6. Emphysema

_____ 7. Other condition

_____

_____

_____

Symptoms

_____ 8. Persistent cough

_____ 9. Chest pains

_____ 10. Difficult or labored breathing

_____ 11. Wheezing or asthma

_____ 12. Productive cough (phlegm, sputum)

_____ 13. Coughing up blood

_____ 14. Other symptoms

_____

A22. Cardiovascular system
Symptoms or diagnosed conditions
Year of occurrence or diagnosis

_____ 1. Heart attack

_____ 2. Heart disease

_____ 3. Rapid or irregular heartbeat

_____ 4. Heart murmur

_____ 5. Swollen feet or ankles

_____ 6. High blood pressure

_____ 7. Stroke

_____ 8. Low blood pressure

_____ 9. Hardening of the arteries

_____ 10. Vasculitis

_____ 11. Thrombophlebitis

_____ 12. Other disease of veins or arteries

_____ 13. Other conditions

_____

_____

_____

A23. Blood
Diagnosed conditions
Year of occurrence or diagnosis

———— 1. ITP

———— 2. Anemia

———— 3. Infectious
mononucleosis

———— 4. Malaria

———— 5. Condition of spleen

———— 6. Dialysis or pheresis
(reason?)

———— 7. Abnormal blood count

———— 8. Blood transfusion

———— 9. Coagulation or clotting
disorder

———— 10. Other conditions

_____

_____

_____

A24. Digestive
Diagnosed conditions
Year of occurrence or diagnosis

———— 1. Gallstones

———— 2. Ulcers—any site

———— 3. Hepatitis

———— 4. Jaundice

———— 5. Cirrhosis of liver

———— 6. Other conditions of
liver or pancreas

———— 7. Esophageal atresia

———— 8. Frequent nausea
or vomiting

———— 9. Chronic indigestion

———— 10. Colic or abdominal
cramps

———— 11. Frequent diarrhea

———— 12. Frequent constipation

———— 13. Loss of appetite

———— 14. Loss of weight

———— 15. Alcohol or food
intolerance

———— 16. Other symptoms

_____

_____

A25. Urinary tract
Diagnosed conditions
Year of occurrence or diagnosis   *Symptoms*

_____ 1. Kidney condition   _____ 4. Frequent or painful urination

_____ 2. Bladder disease   _____ 5. Blood in urine

_____ 3. Protein in urine   _____ 6. Other symptoms

_____ _____

A26. Endocrine/glandular system
Symptoms or diagnosed conditions
Year of occurrence or diagnosis

_____ 1. Diabetes   _____ 5. Hypoglycemia

_____ 2. Thyroid condition   _____ 6. Other

_____ 3. Any hormonal   _____
              condition

_____ 4. Excessive sweating   _____

A27. Skin
Diagnosed conditions
Year of occurrence or diagnosis

_____ 1. Psoriasis

_____ 2. Eczema

_____ 3. Dermatitis

Symptoms

_____ 4. Unusual rashes   _____ 10. Easy or spontaneous
                                                     bruising

_____ 5. Red, scaly, dry, or   _____ 11. Small, round purple
              itching skin   or red spots

_____ 6. Unusual acne   _____ 12. Other symptoms

_____ 7. Hives or boils   _____

_____ 8. Unusual flushing   _____

_____ 9. Patches of greater or
              less pigmentation   _____

A28. Immune system
Symptoms or diagnosed conditions
Year of occurrence or diagnosis

————   1. Hay fever

————   2. Asthma

————   3. Food allergies

————   4. Allergic dermatitis
            or skin rashes

————   5. Frequent colds
            or infections

————   6. Chemical intolerance

————   7. Other

————————————————————

A29. Head and neck
Symptoms or diagnosed conditions
Year of occurrence or diagnosis

————   1. Excessively oily or
            brittle hair

————   2. Unusual loss of hair

————   3. Nasal soreness

————   4. Sinus troubles or
            infections

————   5. Excessive salivation

————   6. Prolonged sore throat

————   7. Dry throat

————   8. Difficulty in
            swallowing

————   9. Unusual taste in
            mouth (e.g., metal,
            garlic)

————   10. Excessive dental
            cavities

————   11. Excessive tooth loss
            (other than baby
            teeth)

————   12. Swollen or sore gums

————   13. Eyes—red, itchy, watery,
             sore, dry, inflamed, other
             (specify)

————————————————————

————————————————————

————   14. Blurred vision

————   15. Constricted pupils

————   16. Corrective lenses needed

————   17. Cataracts

————   18. Glaucoma

————   19. Ears—itching, pain,
             or discharge

————   20. Head injuries (any
             after effects?)

————————————————————

————   21. Other

————————————————————

A30. Nervous System
Symptoms or diagnosed conditions
Year of occurrence or diagnosis

_____	1.	Epilepsy or seizures	_____ 12.	Anxiety
_____	2.	Frequent headaches	_____ 13.	Depression
_____	3.	Frequent dizziness	_____ 14.	Trouble sleeping (at least once a week lasting six months)
___	4.	Weakness, fatigue		
_____	5.	Lethargy, drowsiness	_____ 15.	Irritability
_____	6.	Decreased sensory perception—smell, taste, hearing, vision, touch	_____ 16.	Hyperactivity
			_____ 17.	Restlessness or trouble sitting still
_____	7.	Color vision (What color is hard to see?)	_____ 18.	Learning disorder
			_____ 19.	Memory or personality changes
_____	8.	Trouble discriminating colors in dim light	_____ 20.	Frequent nightmares
			_____ 21.	Meningitis
_____	9.	Numbness, tingling, prickling, other sensations on skin	_____ 22.	Peripheral neuropathy
			_____ 23.	Other
_____	10.	Tremors, cramps, spasms		
_____	11.	Problems with balance, coordination, reaction time, clumsiness		

A31. Muscles and bones
Symptoms or diagnosed conditions
Year of occurrence or diagnosis

_____	1.	Arthritis/rheumatism	_____ 4.	Broken bones
_____	2.	Limb pain, hand or foot	_____ 5.	Numbness, weakness in arms or legs
_____	3.	Stiffness in joints	_____ 6.	Leg cramps

_____ 7. Muscular dystrophy   _____ 10. Other

_____ 8. Multiple sclerosis

_____

_____ 9. Other muscle or
              bone pain

_____

A32. Other
Symptoms or diagnosed conditions
Year of occurrence or diagnosis

_____ 1. Cancer   _____ 8. Unexplained loss or
          What sites? _____   gain in weight

                                           _____ 9. Twenty pounds over-
_____   weight or underweight

_____ 2. Leukemia
                                          _____ 10. Frequently feel
_____ 3. Hodgkin's disease   warmer or colder
                                          than others
_____ 4. Any metabolic
          disorder   _____ 11. Cysts
          Specify:_____

                                           _____ 12. Accidents that required
_____   medical care (including
                                          athletic injuries)
_____ 5. Fever

                                           _____ 13. Serious infections
_____ 6. Chills   What site?_____

_____ 7. Other conditions or
          complaints   _____

                                           _____ 14. Other
_____

_____   _____

                                           _____

A33. Female
Diagnosed conditions
Year of occurrence or diagnosis

_____ 1. Menopause   _____ 4. Female hormones
                                           (estrogen) prescribed
_____ 2. Irregular periods

                                           _____ 5. Disorder of cervix
_____ 3. Premenstrual syn-
          drome   _____ 6. Disorder of uterus

111

| | 7. Disorder of ovaries | | 10. Other |

         7. Disorder of ovaries   10. Other

         8. Venereal disease

         9. Infertility

A33. Male
Diagnosed conditions
Year of occurrence or diagnosis

         1. Sterility   4. Venereal disease

         2. Abnormal sperm count   5. Other

         3. Sexual disturbances or problems

A34. *Major medications*
Please indicate any prescribed medication you have ever taken regularly or taken at onset of symptoms. Include pain relievers only if taken regularly for three months or more; do not include antibiotics for minor infections unless infections are recurrent and antibiotics are used at each onset. Do include antiparasitic agents. Do include medications taken for more than one month for preventive purposes (such as antimalarials or antituberculosis drugs). Indicate approximate years you took them, and especially list all those you take regularly now.

A35. Radiation history: approximate number and years of X rays
1. Screening (chest, mammography, dental)

2. Diagnostic (what body part, how many, when)

3. Therapeutic radiation (what type, what underlying condition, how many treatments, when)

A36. How do you rate your general health?
- ☐ 1. Poor
- ☐ 2. Fair
- ☐ 3. Average
- ☐ 4. Better than average
- ☐ 5. Excellent

A37. Have there been any changes in your health in the past five years? Examples: gradual improvement or decline in health, seasonal variations, any change (better or worse) when you leave the area for a while.

_____

_____

A38. Are there any other health complaints you are concerned about?

_____

_____

_____

Section B. Occupation and Life-Style

This section includes a summary of all jobs held since age sixteen and detailed information for jobs held within the past five years (one form per job). The administrator of the survey will provide extra sheets if needed.

Summary of Occupations since Age Sixteen

Job 1 (present job)
  Place of employment_____

  Department_____

  What years employed? _____

  Was a physical required?_____

Job 2 (previous job)
  Place of employment _____

  Department _____

  What years employed? _____

  Was a physical required?_____

113

Job 3
    Place of employment_____

    Department _____

    What years employed?_____

    Was a physical required?_____

Job 4
    Place of employment _____

    Department _____

    What years employed?_____

    Was a physical required?_____

Job 5
    Place of employment_____

    Department_____

    What years employed? _____

    Was a physical required?_____

Job 6
    Place of employment _____

    Department _____

    What years employed?_____

    Was a physical required? _____

Job 7
    Place of employment _____

    Department_____

    What years employed?_____

    Was a physical required?_____

Job 8
    Place of employment _____

114

Department _____

What years employed? _____

Was a physical required? _____

Job 9
  Place of employment _____

Department _____

What years employed? _____

Was a physical required? _____

Job 10
  Place of employment _____

Department _____

What years employed? _____

Was a physical required? _____

Occupational Information

Please answer this question for each job held during the past five years, including self-employment, lasting six months or more.

Job _____ (from 19____ to 19____)

  B1. Place of employment

  _____

  B2. Main activity of company or organization

  _____

  B3. Relevant activities or products

  _____

  B4. If industrial, production process used

  _____

B5. Describe the type of place usually worked
- ☐ 1. Factory or plant
- ☐ 2. Laboratory
- ☐ 3. Vehicle
- ☐ 4. Warehouse
- ☐ 5. Outdoors
- ☐ 6. Office
- ☐ 7. Restaurant or hotel
- ☐ 8. Other

_____

B6. Department

_____

B7. Specific tasks and materials used

_____

B8. Did you ever have to replace someone else or have to be replaced? If so, how often?

_____

B9. Describe work surroundings (number of people, noise, temperature, machines)

_____

B10. Were there dust, fumes, smoke, gases? If so, what specifically, including cigarette smoke?

_____

B11. Did you work with oils, solvents, acids, detergents? If so, what specifically?

_____

B12. Did your job involve exposure to X rays or microwaves? If so, what was their function?

_____

B13. Did you have to wear protective equipment? If so, what and why?

_____

B14. Did this job have a bad effect on your physical health? If so, how or why?

_____

B15. Was there anything you did not like to do?

_____

B16. What is the source of your drinking water at work?

_____

B17. Did any of those performing the same job have a common complaint(s) or illness?

_____

Repeat B1–B17 for each job held during the past five years.

B18. To your knowledge, are you now or have you ever been frequently exposed to any of the following chemicals at work? Give approximate inclusive dates for frequent exposures.

Job Number (see Summary of Occupations) and Inclusive Years of Exposure

1. Acrylonitrile _____

2. Arsenic _____

3. Asbestos _____

4. Benzene _____

5. Beryllium _____

6. Bis(chloromethyl)ether _____

7. Ceramic dust or talc _____

8. Coal tar pitch, volatiles _____

9. Oils, asphalt _____

10. Chemical fertilizers _____

11. Coke oven emissions _____

12. Dyes _____

13. Lacquers, varnishes _____

14. Fiberglass _____

15. Cotton, textile, wood, grain, or metal dust _____

16. Paints, glues _____

17. Organic solvents, paint thinners _____

18. Isopropyl oils _____

19. Other petroleum products _____

20. Radioisotopes or radio-active materials _____

21. Insecticides, pesticides _____

22. Herbicides, fungicides _____

23. Chromium or chromates _____

B19. Have you ever been told you have an occupationally related disease or reaction? If yes, please indicate person, year recognized, and agent if known (examples: allergic dermatitis, pneumoconiosis or lung disease, neurological effects)

_____

_____

_____

B20. Indicate which of the following substances you have used frequently, perhaps in your hobby or around the house.

☐ 1. Plastics	☐ 16. Fixatives
☐ 2. Metals	☐ 17. Oil paints
☐ 3. Clay	☐ 18. Acrylic paints
☐ 4. Wood	☐ 19. Alkyd paints
☐ 5. Paper	☐ 20. Epoxy paints
☐ 6. Stone	☐ 21. Aerosol or spray paints
☐ 7. Glazes	☐ 22. Lacquer, varnish
☐ 8. Enamels	☐ 23. Acid, caustics
☐ 9. Pastels	☐ 24. Solvents—turpentine, paint thinner, paint removers, other solvents
☐ 10. Dyes	
☐ 11. Plaster	☐ 25. Glues, adhesives, resins
☐ 12. Pigments	☐ 26. Photography chemicals
☐ 13. Feathers	☐ 27. Pesticides, insecticides, fungicides, herbicides, fumigants
☐ 14. Wax	
☐ 15. Glass	

Neighborhood Description

B21. Water

1. Does your water ever taste or smell unusual?_____

2. Is it corrosive or does it discolor cooking utensils or pipes? _____

3. Is it hard?_____

4. Does it leave a film or residue?_____

5. Do you use a water softener? _____

6. Do you use a charcoal filter or ion exchanger?_____

7. Do you add anything to soften your water? _____

B22. What is the general quality of air in your neighborhood?

☐ 1. Clear
☐ 2. Haze
☐ 3. Light smog
☐ 4. Moderate smog
☐ 5. Heavy smog
☐ 6. Occasional dust or smoke

☐ 7. Frequent dust or smoke
☐ 8. Occasional chemical smell
☐ 9. Frequent chemical smell
☐ 10. Other (description)

_____

B23. Do you know of or suspect a specific source of neighborhood pollution or contamination?

_____

_____

B24. Have you noticed any other "environmental clues" you think may be relevant (clusters of dead trees, large barren patches, oil sheen on puddles, fish kills, honeybee kills, unusual frequency of sick pets or livestock), or do you have any other pertinent information?

_____

_____

_____

B25. Indoor pollution description: Is the household regularly exposed to any of the following?

1. Tobacco smoke
   ☐ Never
   ☐ Occasionally/seasonally
   ☐ Frequently

2. Unvented gas space heater
   - ☐ Never
   - ☐ Occasionally/seasonally
   - ☐ Frequently
3. Gas stove
   - ☐ Never
   - ☐ Occasionally/seasonally
   - ☐ Frequently
4. Woodburning or coal-burning stove
   - ☐ Never
   - ☐ Occasionally/seasonally
   - ☐ Frequently

5. Floor wax, furniture polish, oven clean
   - ☐ Never
   - ☐ Occasionally/seasonally
   - ☐ Frequently
6. Roach spray, insecticides, foggers
   - ☐ Never
   - ☐ Occasionally/seasonally
   - ☐ Frequently
7. Anything else? Specify

_____

Lifestyle Description

B26. Is anyone in the family on a special or restricted diet? If yes, what type and why?

_____

_____

_____

B27. Cigarettes

_____ 1. Number smoked per day   _____ 3. Year quit

_____ 2. Year begun   _____ 4. Did you inhale?

B28. Cigars

_____ 1. Number smoked per day   _____ 3. Year quit

_____ 2. Year begun   _____ 4. Did you inhale?

B29. Chewing or smokeless tobacco

_____ 1. Packs or ounces chewed per day _____ 3. Year quit

_____ 2. Year begun   _____ 4. Did you swallow?

B30. Snuff

_____ 1. Number of dips per day

_____ 2. Year begun

_____ 3. Year quit

B31. Pipe

_____ 1. Number smoked per day   _____ 3. Year quit

_____ 2. Year begun   _____ 4. Did you inhale?

B32. Recreational drugs (number used per week)

_____ 1. Amphetamines (stimulants)   _____ 4. Other

_____ 2. Barbiturates   _____

_____ 3. Marijuana   _____

B33. Alcoholic beverages (number per week)

_____ 1. Beer

_____ 2. Wine

_____ 3. Mixed drinks

Section C. Reproductive History

All women answer this section; answer all questions that apply.

C1. Are you currently pregnant?
   ☐ Yes
   ☐ No
   ☐ Don't know

C2. Have you ever been pregnant?
   ☐ Yes
   ☐ No
   ☐ Don't know

C3. Has a doctor ever advised you not to become pregnant (again)?
   ☐ Yes
   ☐ No
   ☐ Don't know
   If yes, what was the doctor's reason for this?

_____

C4. Have you ever been told you are sterile or have reached menopause?
   ☐ Sterile
   ☐ Menopause
   ☐ No
   If so, year?_____

C5. Are you currently using or have you used some birth control method?
- ☐ 1. Pill
- ☐ 2. Foam, cream, or jelly
- ☐ 3. IUD
- ☐ 4. Sterile—wife
- ☐ 5. Sterile—husband
- ☐ 6. Abortion
- ☐ 7. Other (please specify)

_____
- ☐ 8. Hysterectomy/vasectomy

C6. Have you ever wanted to become pregnant but been physically unable?
- ☐ Yes
- ☐ No
- ☐ Don't know

C7. Have you ever seen a doctor because you had trouble getting pregnant?
- ☐ Yes
- ☐ No

If yes, when? _____

What was the doctor's diagnosis?
- ☐ Anatomical defect
- ☐ Hormonal/glandular
- ☐ No reported abnormality
- ☐ Other (specify)

_____

C8. Has your husband ever seen a doctor because you had trouble getting pregnant?
- ☐ Yes
- ☐ No
- ☐ Don't know

If yes, when? _____

What was the doctor's diagnosis?
- ☐ Anatomical defect
- ☐ Hormonal/glandular
- ☐ Low sperm count
- ☐ Impotence
- ☐ No reported abnormality
- ☐ Other (specify)

_____

C9. How many times all together have you been pregnant? Please be sure to include all pregnancies that ended in a live birth, a miscarriage, a stillbirth, or an induced abortion.

_____

C10. How many babies have been born to you, including any who died after birth?

_____

122

Stop here if there have been no pregnancies. Continue if there was a pregnancy, regardless of outcome. Extra sheets provided by the survey administrator may be used for more babies.

Answer for each baby:	First	Second	Third

C11. Was your baby a boy or a girl? _____ _____ _____

C12. In what year did each pregnancy end? _____ _____ _____

C13. Did this pregnancy result in

	First	Second	Third
1. Normal vaginal birth	☐	☐	☐
2. Cesarean	☐	☐	☐
3. Stillbirth	☐	☐	☐
4. Abortion (induced)	☐	☐	☐
5. Twins, both live	☐	☐	☐
6. Twins, one live, one stillborn	☐	☐	☐
7. Other multiple outcome	☐	☐	☐
8. Tubal pregnancy	☐	☐	☐
9. Low birth-weight baby (less than 5½ pounds or 2500 grams)	☐	☐	☐
10. Premature birth (less than thirty-seven weeks)	☐	☐	☐
11. Miscarriage	☐	☐	☐
How long had you been pregnant at the time of the miscarriage?	_____	_____	_____

C14. Did your baby/babies have any condition at birth or apparent shortly afterward that involved (please specify):

	First	Second	Third
1. Extremities (arms, legs, hands, feet)	☐	☐	☐
2. Skin rashes or darkened skin	☐	☐	☐
3. Moles/birthmarks	☐	☐	☐
4. Head—molding	☐	☐	☐
5. Eyes—abnormalities	☐	☐	☐
6. Lips—cleft, other	☐	☐	☐
7. Gums—cleft, born with teeth	☐	☐	☐
8. Palate—cleft, other	☐	☐	☐
9. Other facial features	☐	☐	☐
10. Ears	☐	☐	☐
11. Thorax—large, small	☐	☐	☐
12. Lungs—not fully inflated	☐	☐	☐
difficulty breathing	☐	☐	☐

13.	Heart—abnormal rhythm or rate	☐	☐	☐
	murmur	☐	☐	☐
	valve defect	☐	☐	☐
	other	☐	☐	☐
14.	Liver—jaundice	☐	☐	☐
	other	☐	☐	☐
15.	Spleen	☐	☐	☐
16.	Kidneys	☐	☐	☐
17.	Skeletal—muscles	☐	☐	☐
	bones	☐	☐	☐
	joints	☐	☐	☐
18.	Stomach	☐	☐	☐
19.	Intestines	☐	☐	☐
20.	Throat	☐	☐	☐
21.	Genitals—male	☐	☐	☐
	female	☐	☐	☐
22.	Brain—cerebral palsy, other	☐	☐	☐
	spinal	☐	☐	☐
	other nervous system condition	☐	☐	☐
	mental condition	☐	☐	☐
23.	Reflexes—abnormal	☐	☐	☐
24.	Metabolic disorder	☐	☐	☐
25.	Chromosomal disorder	☐	☐	☐
26.	Any other condition apparent or occurring at birth			

C15. Did any baby require extra time in the hospital after delivery?_____
If so, why?

_____

Section D. Children's Health

Please answer each question for each child. "Children" includes persons through eighteen years of age. Answer as appropriate for the age of the child.

Household member number, to match section A_____

D1. Sex and present age of child

_____

D2. In general, would you say your child's health is excellent, good, fair, or poor?

_____

D3. Does your child seem less healthy than other children his/her age?
   ☐ Yes
   ☐ No
   ☐ Don't know

D4. Does your child seem to resist illness well?
   ☐ Yes
   ☐ No
   ☐ Intermediate

D5. Has your child ever been seriously ill? Specify:

_____

What year was this diagnosed? _____

D6. Does health limit this child in any way from doing what he/she wants to do?
   ☐ Yes
   ☐ No
   ☐ Don't know

   Specify: _____

   _____

D7. Does health limit the amount or kind of ordinary play he/she can do?

   _____

   Specify: _____

   _____

D8. Does health limit the kind or amount of vigorous or strenuous activities he/she can do?

   _____

   Specify: _____

   _____

D9. In the past year, has your child seemed to be:
   ☐ 1. Bothered by nervousness or "nerves"   ☐ 5. Unable to concentrate
   ☐ 2. Anxious or worried   ☐ 6. Hyperactive
   ☐ 3. Restless or impatient   ☐ 7. Losing interest in things
   ☐ 4. Depressed or moody   ☐ 8. Doing worse in school or sports

D10. During the past year has your child gotten along well with:
    ☐ 1. Other children
    ☐ 2. The family
    ☐ 3. Teachers and classmates

D11. Do you feel your child has developed normally during
    ☐ 1. 0–4 years of age
    ☐ 2. 5–16 years of age

D12. Does your child have any learning or reading disorder that requires special attention? Specify

_____

_____

D13. In the past year, has your child been doing as well academically in school as you think he/she should or as he/she has done in the past?

_____

_____

D14. Does your child have any other conditions that might require special attention or adaptation? Specify

_____

_____

_____

D15. Does your child require regular or frequent medication, injections, or supplements of any sort other than children's aspirin or vitamins? Specify reason and treatment.

_____

_____

_____

D16. Is or was your child's diet limited by
    ☐ 1. Allergies   ☐ 4. Other
    ☐ 2. Metabolic condition
    ☐ 3. Preference   _____

D17. Are there any other complaints or conditions that arise in your child more often than you think they should, or anything you think is not normal? Specify (refer if needed to the checklist in the first section).

_____

_____

_____

D18. Did (does) your child do well in
    ☐ 1. Nursery school   ☐ 3. Preschool
    ☐ 2. Day care   ☐ 4. Kindergarten

D19. Were (are) his/her height and weight normal? If not, specify how not.

_____

_____

D20. Was (is) his/her mental development normal? If not, specify.

_____

_____

D21. Have any conditions present at birth been resolved or permanently corrected? Specify (refer to reproductive history section).

_____

_____

_____

D22. Are there any other problems or conditions that you would like to detail?

_____

_____

_____

Questions Concerning the Administration of This Questionnaire

1. Time it took to complete _____

2. Were any questions

	Section	Question	Part	Why
Too technical?	_____	_____	_____	_____
Confusing?	_____	_____	_____	_____
Other?	_____	___ ___	_ _ ___	_____

3. Do you think an interviewer, if present, inhibited your response to any question?
   ☐ Yes
   ☐ Somewhat
   ☐ No

4. Were there questions you think would be answered more honestly in general without an interviewer present?
   ☐ Reproductive history ☐ Other
   ☐ Amount smoked
   ☐ Amount drunk _____
   ☐ Use of recreational drugs

5. Any other comments will be appreciated.

Attach a blank sheet if more space is required for any given answer. (Indicate section, question, and person responding)

Question Discussion

Section A. Family Description and General Health

The issue of confidentiality has been discussed; your experimental design determines whether you need to know the exact location of every household. Since you are collecting individual cases within households, you will need an identification number (for tabulation purposes) for *each person* as well as for each household.

A1. Some traits have definite racial or cultural associations.

A2. The type of neighborhood will describe in part such factors as pollution, pesticide use, and water source. This is not necessary if the entire sample is the same.

A3. Neighborhood quality can be assessed by income; income also correlates with general awareness of environmental issues, personal health care, and many other things.

A4. A general descriptive element.

A5. This question is necessary unless exposure is known to be less than one year.

A6. Identifies people who have lived in more than one place within the community.

A7. Necessary to determine sample size.

A8–9. Necessary if you want to know whether moderate or long-term exposures might have already contributed to death rates. The second part (A9) may identify exposed persons who have been affected and moved away. The five-year limit is arbitrary; a longer time period may pick up earlier deaths.

A10. Is everyone in the community using the same water source? If waterborne exposure is suspected, is anyone using bottled water? (Later you might ask how long they used each water source.)

A11–15. Minimally, you will need to know the age, sex, height, weight, and educational level of each person.

A16–19. Possibly of interest in situations of herbicide application (Agent Orange, for example). This does not include members of the Reserves.

A20. Since many diseases run in families, this question pertains to the respondents (and spouses, if applicable) and to other family members who do not live in the household and therefore probably were not exposed.

As a rule of thumb, if any condition occurs in three
or more first-degree relatives of a respondent, you may
decide to disregard that condition if it also appears
in the respondent. In this way you will obtain a conservative estimate, since you will not be counting
predisposition for a particular condition even though
it may have been environmentally triggered. You
will still be counting any symptom that does not appear
to run in the family. However, many surveys do not
assess family history at all; if you leave it out, you will
then be counting environmentally triggered conditions
to which a person is especially vulnerable (an equally
valid measurement anyway). If you do use this question,
by correlating family conditions with environmentally
triggered systems, you may identify high-risk groups
and thus provide an early warning system. On the whole,
we recommend leaving this question in.

A21–33. For the preliminary survey you will want to assess
effects on all organ systems. Even for a condensed questionnaire, health effects are the core of your entire
survey, so while you initially approach your survey with
the idea of measuring incidence for only a few specific
conditions, remember that people can respond in
different ways to the same chemical. By conducting a
thorough survey from the start, you will avoid having
to go back to ask about other conditions you were not
aware of at first.

A34. This question asks about major medications taken
regularly or continually. Many drugs have adverse side
effects, and you cannot hope to pick up all such effects,
but drugs taken in large amounts should be recorded
here.

Section B. Occupation and Life-style

Summary
of Occupa-
tions and
B1–19. Complete occupational histories are required in any
good epidemiologic study, owing to the large number
of people with occupational exposures to toxic substances. If you have recently seen a sudden onset of

acute symptoms, you will still need to ascertain current jobs to rule out an uneven employment pattern. Even if you know exactly what the chemical in question is and where it comes from, occupational exposures may contribute to the appearance and severity of symptoms. If you do not know whether there is a health problem or know there is a problem but not where it is coming from, you will need a complete job history (jobs beginning with age eighteen and lasting six months) plus the more detailed questions (B1–17) on recent jobs. If this job required a physical examination, there may be a doctor's record of it, and thus you may be able to verify past health status.

B20.   Toxic exposures from arts and crafts are often underestimated.

B21.   Water treatment or characteristics may vary between households.

B22.   You may be able to answer this for the entire community. The answer is subjective and does not indicate frequency. Pollution may be regarded as more serious by persons who are adversely affected by it.

B23.   A "discovery" question that may be more appropriate as an issue discussed at a group meeting.

B24.   Same comment, but this depends more on individual observation.

B25.   This is included to underline the importance of indoor pollution, and it can also indicate exposures that can be many times more toxic than outdoor pollution. Gas heaters and woodburning stoves can be particularly polluting, but their use may be consistent between your groups. Even so, we recommend leaving this question in.

Section C. Reproductive History

C1–10.   The minimum core of questions that should be asked of all women of reproductive age. We know much less about the effect of chemicals on reproductive outcomes, so we probably underestimate the incidence of reproductive effects.

Section D. Children's Health

We believe this section should be used intact, since there are no reference values for general incidence of the characteristics queried. It will be of absolutely no value to assess the children of your community without assessing the children of a control community just as carefully. What if 20 percent of the children in your randomly selected households of 20 percent of *all* the children in your study group are hyperactive? What if one-third of them have allergies? The same might be true of unexposed communities. You might find discussions of the incidence of certain kinds of learning disabilities, but since we are still discovering how to measure them, the rates are not accurate. Your school board, even if willing to help, can at best give you only a vague idea of the incidence of dyslexia or the number in remedial classes or similar statistics. These rates are entirely dependent on testing for them in public schools, and their severity (or degree of correction) depends on the quality of corrective education. In a similar vein, pediatricians will not have a feeling for incidence rates of health problems, because they see only a portion of the affected children and even fewer of the unaffected. Thus you will be shortchanging your children if you have no adequate control group of unexposed children with which to compare them.

Coding the Answers for the Tabulation Forms

By coding you reduce a vast amount of information to a shorthand or code in which each possible answer to a multiple choice question is replaced by a number. Thus the answer to question A2 (type of neighborhood), which offers five choices, is coded as a number between 1 and 5. Dates will be coded as the last two digits of the year. Codes are often listed 01 to 99 merely to reserve enough spaces for each digit, not because there are 99 possible responses. The format used here describes how to code every digit; for example, for the identification numbers in section A, the first three digits represent the household number, the next two represent the person in the household, and the last digit is the code for control or exposed. On a computer card, should you be able to process your information this way, this answer occupies only six spaces on the card. Exactly how to formulate punch cards and read them into a computer is not described here, since anyone who has the facilities to do this will also have the expertise. Figure 6.1 shows a tabulation form.

Identification number	Address

A	1	2	3	4	5	6	7	8	9	
	10	11	12	13	14	15	16	17	18	19

	20							Other symptoms
	21 Lung							
	22 Cardiovascular							
	23 Blood							
	24 Digestive							
	25 Urinary							
	26 Endocrine							
	27 Skin							
	28 Immune							
	29 Head and Neck							
	30 Nervous System							
	31 Muscles, bones							
	32 Other					Cancer:		
	33 Male			33 Female				
	34							
	35						36	
	37				38			

B	Occupational summary:				
	18	19	20		
	21	22	23	24	25
	26	27	28	29	
	30	31	32	33	

C	1	2	3	4	5	6	7	8	9	10
	11	12	13	14	15					

D	1	2	3	4	5	6	7	8	9	10
	11	12	13	14	15	16	17	18	19	20
	21	22								

Figure 6.1 A Tabulation Form

Section A. Family Description and General Health

Identification number 001–999, one number per person, *or* 001–999, number per household/01–99 number of each person within each household, to coordinate residence; 1 = control, 2 = exposed, or C, H, M, L for control, high, medium, low exposures. Example: 023/3/M = twenty-third household, third member, medium exposure group or stratum.

A1. Race: 1–6
A2. Neighborhood: 1–5
A3. Income: 1–5
A4. Housing: 1–3
A5. Present address: 19___ (give last two digits of year)
A6. Year moved to community: 19___
A7. Number of regular household members
A8. Recent death? 1 = yes, 2 = no. If yes, write in who and cause of death
A9. Other departure? 1 = yes, 2 = no. If yes, write in who and why
A10. Water source: 1–4
A11. Age
A12. Sex: 1 = male, 2 = female
A13. Height in inches
A14. Weight in pounds
A15. Education: 12 = high school, 16 = college, etc.
A16. Service: 1–5
A17. Year entered 19___
A18. Year left 19___
A19. Tour: 1–6
A20. All positive responses, such as 1p, 12d, 21ee, etc.
A21–33. In each box, write diagnosis or symptom number and year indicated (last two digits). Write in what other symptoms or conditions and cancer site. Answer A33 for male or female as appropriate. Example: for A22: 02 78; 09–76.
A34. Write in medications
A35. Copy radiation history
A36. General health: 1–5
A37–38. Summarize response

Section B. Occupation and Life-style

Occupational summary: Summarize, for example as: teacher/administrator 1970–83 (arts and craft supplies). Miscellaneous clerical jobs 1960–80 (cigarette smoke). Trucker/mechanic 1940–80, retired (degreasers, solvents). Indicate potential responses from B1–17, to be analyzed in more detail separately. Indicate major employer also: operator/Able Chemical Company 1965–82 (pesticides, respirator required). This requires a judgment on the part of the tabulator, but key exposures and major jobs noted here should be sufficient until a more thorough occupational analysis needs to be made.

B18.   Job/number
B19.   Occupational disease?
B20.   Any positive numbers
B21.   Water: 1–7 (may be more than one affirmative answer)
B22.   Air: 1–10 (may be more than one affirmative answer)
B23–24. Summarize response
B25.   Indoor air: 1–7; never = 1, occasionally = 2, frequently = 3
B27–31. Smoking: number/year begun 19___/year quit 19___
B32.   Number/how many per week
B33.   Number/how many per week

Section C. Reproductive History

C1–3. 1 = yes, 2 = no, 3 = don't know
C4.   1 = sterile, 2 = menopause (year), 3 = no/year
C5.   Birth control: 1–8/number for past/number for present
C6.   1 = yes, 2 = no, 3 = don't know
C7.   1 = yes, 2 = no/year/ 3 = anatomical, 4 = hormonal, 5 = no abnormality, 6 = other (what?)
C8.   1 = yes, 2 = no, 3 = don't know, 4 = anatomical, 5 = hormonal, 6 = sperm count, 7 = impotence, 8 = no abnormality, 9 = other (what?)
C9.   Pregnancies: number
C10.   Births: number
C11.   Birth number/1 = boy, 2 = girl
C12.   Write years of pregnancies (63, 65, 66, 68, 71, for example)
C13.   Pregnancy number/1–9
C14.   Baby number/defect(s) (1–26)
C15.   Baby number/reason (3/jaundice, for example)

Section D. Children's Health

D1.   Age/1 = boy, 2 = girl/household member number should agree with section A
D2.   1 = excellent, 2 = good, 3 = fair, 4 = poor
D3.   1 = yes, 2 = no, 3 = don't know
D4.   1 = yes, 2 = no, 3 = intermediate
D5.   What/year
D6.   1 = yes, 2 = no, 3 = don't know
D7–8. 1 = yes, 2 = no/what
D9.   1–8 (may be more than one answer)
D10.   1–3 (indicate a negative response)

D11.   1–2 (indicate a negative respone)
D12–15. 1 = yes, 2 = no
D16.   1–4 (indicate a negative response)
D17.   1 = yes, 2 = no
D18.   1–4 (indicate a negative response)
D19–20. Summarize responses

Lots of Information—
What to Do with It
Statistics for Nonstatisticians

Michael J. Scott
Barbara L. Harper

he next step, tabulation, consists simply of adding up the number of responses to a question or how many choices were marked. Initial totals will tell you some basic things about the two groups you have surveyed, such as how many people are in each age group, how many are male and how many female, and what organ systems are most affected. Simple comparisons can be made by going back through the tabulation forms (or by drawing from your data base if you have the information on a computer) and asking questions such as how many females have a particular condition or when did the symptoms start to appear. Each question of this kind generates four groups—variable A (yes or no) crossed with variable B (yes or no). Thus, every time you wish to examine a different factor you must go back through the tabulation forms and read the answers for the new set of factors. This is obviously a time-consuming process, but educated guesses about which factors to use to follow significant health effects should allow you to avoid many dead ends. To determine if any difference you may see between your two groups is "real" (i.e., statistically convincing to health authorities), you can apply some simple tests to see if the number of cases of something you observe is different than you would normally expect to see. The number you derive from this tells you how sure you can be that the difference you see between the exposed and unexposed groups is not due just to chance or natural variation. We have assumed that any event that is expected to occur less than 10 percent of the time may be significant. Comparing your results with a national or regional average requires different, but still simple, calculations. Other basic questions are also discussed: How does normal variation in the background rate affect the ability to detect increases? If there really is a difference, how sure can I be of detecting it? Will I be able to detect a twofold increase or a fourfold increase? If I have an idea of what the normal rate for a particular condition is, how many exposed persons do I need to survey to detect a reasonable increase in that condition? How does sample size (the number of persons surveyed) affect the sensitivity of the study? What chance is there of my concluding that a difference exists between my two groups when it really does not? Though some calculations may be necessary, tables are provided to help you make some of the decisions.

This chapter will assist you in tabulating your results and organizing them so they can be easily understood. By using many examples based on the questionnaire, we will introduce the concept of comparing results between two groups and determining by simple numerical methods whether there is a real difference.

Tabulating Your Answers and Presenting Your Results
Using the tabulation form in the previous chapter (fig. 6.1), you will have coded all the answers from the survey and reduced the amount of paperwork to one page for each person.

The first type of question in the questionnaire is simple multiple choice. Question 1, for example, has a one-digit answer for race and will be tallied as the number of persons choosing each answer, giving you a racial profile for your communities. Comparing the exposed and unexposed communities will show you if they are similar in racial makeup, which they should be if you have selected your control group correctly. Questions A2, A3, and A4 also describe the community and should be similar for both communities; affluent suburbs are not proper control groups for poor rural areas. The total in question A7 is your sample size and should correspond to the number of completed tabulation forms you have. Questions A5 and A6 (length of residence) will be important when you need to know if conditions (cancer, for instance) occur only in persons who have lived in the area for ten years or more or occur less fre-

Table 7.1   Example of Numbers of Persons in Various Age Groups

Age Group	Male	Female	Total
0–10	10	12	22
11–20	8	11	19
21–30	15	17	32
31–40	23	25	48
41–50	18	17	35
51–60	8	10	18
61–70	13	16	29
71–80	15	17	32
81 or more	4	6	10
Total	114	131	245

quently in persons of the same age who moved there only a short time ago.

Question A11 will give you the age distribution, or how many people are in each age group. When you are finished tabulating, your results for one community may look like table 7.1. This information can also be presented as a line or bar graph (fig. 7.1). If we make a graph, it becomes apparent that in this example there are two peaks in the age distribution (called a "biomodal distribution"), which might be explained by the presence of many young families plus senior citizens' housing or a large retirement or nursing home. Since you know that the very young and the elderly are especially susceptible to environmental agents, a distribution like this might suggest that you examine in more detail those up to twenty years old and the retirement-age groups. This will also be very important in comparing the age distributions between the two communities. If a community with an older average age has more symptoms than a younger community, you may not be able to compare these two whole groups but rather will have to compare people through twenty years old in one community with people the same age in the other. The same point pertains to examining your results by male versus female.

Specific health effects (A21 through A33) will initially be tallied simply as how many positive responses are recorded for each organ system. Since each person is allowed more than one symptom or condition, the total will be quite large. An initial total for each question will tell you which organ systems are most affected. At this point you can begin to do simple comparisons between number of symptoms reported and other parameters such as water

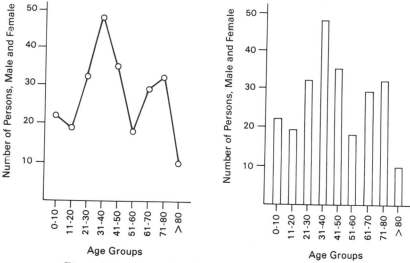

Figure 7.1   **Examples of Line and Bar Graphs of the Number of Persons in Various Age Groups**

source, sex, or age. You will also begin to map your results on a large map or aerial photograph of your community by placing colored pins at the locations of affected persons or households. You may begin to examine specific aspects of your results such as whether males and females are affected in equal proportion, whether males are affected more severely than females, and whether older age groups are more seriously affected. You may also compare your results with year of diagnosis or first occurrence. If you noticed a picture such as that shown in figure 7.2, then you would focus on events that happened in 1980 (new factory, new pesticide, and so on). In other words, the time course of particular acute symptoms may give you valuable clues to the cause. For chronic symptoms or cancer, which have a slowly progressive course and long latency, the cause is obviously long separated from the time of diagnosis. The incidence of conditions that are aggravated little by little over the years will need to be carefully compared with that in the unexposed community. Age in particular is an important parameter, because so many conditions increase in incidence and severity with age. Thus the results from the unexposed community are extremely important in comparing health effects, most of which are expected to occur naturally to some extent and also to increase with age. An example of this might be figure 7.3.

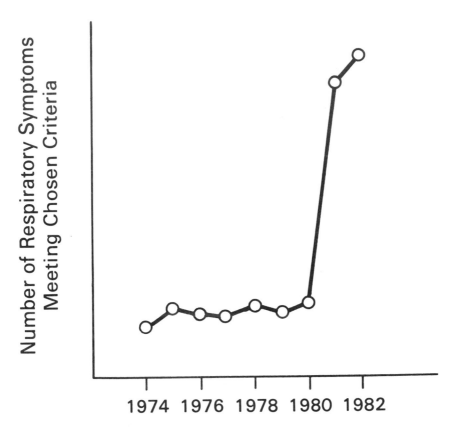

Year of Occurrence or Diagnosis

Figure 7.2   An Example of Disease Incidence by Year of Occurrence

If you did not have information from community A, you would not know whether the rates in community B were elevated. This is particularly important for most health-related conditions, for which there are few local, regional, state, or national data. Cancer statistics (see Appendix) are quite a bit more accurate, and comparing your rates to national rates is discussed below. Birth defect rates, given in the Appendix, also show regional and age-related differences.

Several questions are "open," that is, the person writes in the answer, listing medications, other health complaints, X rays, and so on. These are tabulated as numbers of positive responses, and you will need to compare symptomatic and nonsymptomatic

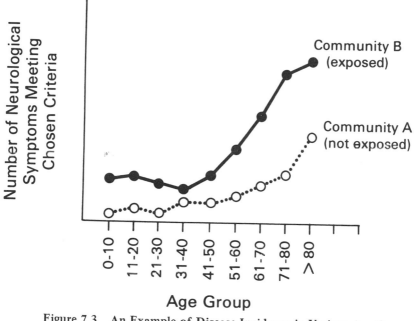

Figure 7.3   An Example of Disease Incidence in Various Age Groups

groups as well as exposed and unexposed groups. It is a circular argument whether initial medical conditions required medication that in turn aggravated other conditions, but you should know the general medication profiles of your various subsamples.

As discussed in the previous chapter, you will need to know if symptoms are related to employment, either as a direct cause or as a contributing factor. For instance, does employment in chemical factory A seem to aggravate respiratory symptoms while employment as a dry cleaner is associated with neurological complaints? This involves many painstaking comparisons and might well bring to light associations that have been overlooked. Questions B18 and B20 (occupational and nonoccupational chemical exposures) might really bring home the point that headaches and solvents go together, for example, and if your survey has no other result than improving ventilation it will have been worthwhile. Likewise, if frequent indoor pollution (B25) plus weatherproofing seems to be correlated with symptoms, your survey might result in local building code changes to require certain air-exchange provisions.

Smoking, drinking, and recreational drugs are of course extremely important variables and should be handled as broad groups after

Table 7.2 Sample Two-by-Two Table

| | Affected | |
	Yes	No
Exposed		
Yes	Group 1	Group 2
No	Group 3	Group 4

tabulating specifics. For example, someone who smokes eight cigarettes a day might go in the one to ten cigarettes a day group. You are entitled to make your own classifications, but if you tabulate exact numbers, you can change your criteria without having to retabulate. General smoking categories might be (1) heavy (over one pack a day), (2) moderate (five to twenty cigarettes a day), (3) light (fewer than five cigarettes a day), (4) quit recently (less than ten years ago), (5) quit more than ten years ago, and (6) never smoked. By looking at the raw numbers you get for cigars, pipes, snuff, and chewing tobacco, you can decide how to divide the respondents into groups (three to five groups per category). Recreational drug use is tabulated by type of drug more than by frequency (anything over once a week is positive for present purposes). Alcohol use is also divided both by type of drink and by frequency, depending on the distribution you find in your results.

When you tabulate reproductive histories and make comparisons, remember that several things other than birth defects are considered to be adverse reproductive effects. Difficulty in getting pregnant may be a sensitive indicator and has in fact been the first clue in several instances of chemical exposure. Spontaneous abortions or miscarriages are also sensitive indicators, as are prematurity and low birth weight.

A discussion of birth defects will introduce the concept of ruling out variables (factors) that do not contribute. Remember that you are not trying to assign a cause for each birth defect, but are trying instead to determine if the rate of birth defects in your community as a whole is elevated with respect to your control community or to regional or national rates, and if common variables can be eliminated, thus leaving environment as a possible contributing cause. Examining one variable at a time means repeatedly dividing both your entire community and the unexposed community in many different ways. For example, you will

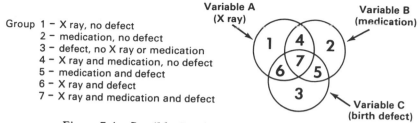

Group 1 – X ray, no defect
      2 – medication, no defect
      3 – defect, no X ray or medication
      4 – X ray and medication, no defect
      5 – medication and defect
      6 – X ray and defect
      7 – X ray and medication and defect

Figure 7.4   Possible Combinations of Three Factors

want to examine both X-ray exposure and medication during pregnancy with respect to birth defects. For each factor you wish to examine you will divide your two communities into appropriate groups, giving you four groups each time: (1) exposed and affected, (2) exposed and not affected, (3) not exposed and affected, and (4) not exposed and not affected (table 7.2).

Additional factors such as medication may be examined separately or may be added to the first two, generating seven groups in our example (fig. 7.4). A fourth variable such as residence or occupation increases the number of possible combinations to fifteen, including single criteria alone, in pairs, in triplets, and all together. Comparing all these groups with one another is called multivariate analysis and will be discussed below.

An alternative to comparing each variable with every other variable at one time is a stepwise analysis that starts with the largest possible number of variables and subdivides little by little, checking for statistical significance at each step so you will know if you are on the right track. For example, in analyzing respiratory problems, divide respondents into heavy smokers, light and moderate smokers, and those who have never smoked or have not smoked for ten years or more. Repeat this process for both exposed and control groups (fig. 7.5).

You will now need to know whether there is any difference between these three groups in incidence of respiratory problems. Methods for making that decision will be discussed shortly. If there is not, lump them all back together and subdivide differently, by male and female, for example. However, if there is no difference between smokers and nonsmokers, the question still remains why nonsmokers are also affected. As you subdivide further and further, thereby defining your affected group more and more specifically, you may find that your "significant" effect disappears. In this

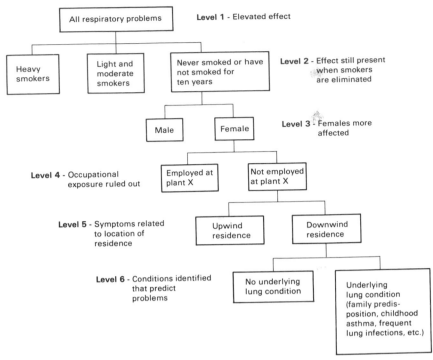

Figure 7.5   Sequential Examination of Possible Contributing Factors

case go back to the level of greatest significance (say females who never smoked—level 3), and compare this incidence rate with that for females who never smoked and were exposed but do not have respiratory problems, and the equivalent females from the control or unexposed population.

Looking for Differences between Your Population and Some Standard

As we pointed out previously, you cannot simply compare the incidence rate for your population with some standard and decide whether the two are different. This is because outcomes naturally vary in subpopulations. Therefore, even though the state average for a certain health problem might be ten in a thousand, your community of one thousand people might easily have anywhere from four to sixteen cases and still be normal. A number of factors contribute to the size of the normal range, and later in this chapter we will talk about some of these factors and what should be considered in designing and analyzing your study.

Since you cannot just compare absolute numbers and rates obtained from your surveys, you will need a couple of statistical tools to help you understand both the implications and the limitations of your data. Two approaches will be presented: one is used in situations where you have data from two populations, either control and exposed or different zones in a stratified population, and the other involves comparing your data with some set of standard health statistics.

Comparing Populations: The Chi-Square Analysis

Basics

Although there are a variety of statistical procedures designed to compare one population with another, one of the most useful and easiest to perform is the chi-square analysis (pronounced ki, to rhyme with pie).

There are two basic concepts associated with chi-square. First, chi-square is structured around some concept of estimating the "expected" value for a population. If we had, for example, a population of 200 people and knew that half of "all people" have brown hair, we would "expect" $200 \times 0.5 = 100$ people in our population to have brown hair. Given this, the second concept is that of differences between what you actually have in your population and what you expected. This difference could be due to natural variation as mentioned earlier, or it could represent a true difference between your population and a "normal" population. For example, your population could have a unique ethnic component, such as a strong Nordic origin, that has caused it not to conform to the "normal" population standard. Chi-square uses these two factors to help you understand your population. By using chi-square you can ask whether two populations are actually the same or whether the difference observed is too big to be attributed to normal variation alone.

Two-by-Two Tables

The easiest way to set up a chi-square analysis is to build a simple table. We will begin with a two-by-two table based on the example given earlier (table 7.3).

A few things to note: this table looks at only two items at a time;

Table 7.3   Sample Two-by-Two Table for Chi-Square Analysis

| | Pulmonary Disease | | Row |
Exposure	Yes	No	Total
Yes	90	210	300
No	85	315	400
Column total	175	525	700

Table 7.4   Determining Expected Frequency of Disease

| | Pulmonary Disease | | Row |
Exposure	Yes	No	Total
Yes	90	210	300
No	85	315	400
Column total	**175**	525	**700**

$$175 \div 700 = 0.25$$

one item is given at the top of the table and the other down the left-hand side; individual columns and rows are totaled, and these subtotals are used to reach the grand total at lower right; and the table consists of the actual number of people who meet a given requirement, not of rates, percentages, or frequencies. The location of the two criteria (exposure and pulmonary disease) is not mandatory (exposure could have been on top), but we suggest that for standardization you keep the health outcome at the top and the exposure criteria on the left side.

This table represents what was actually observed. The next step is to determine what was to be expected had both the exposed and the unexposed populations behaved in the same way with respect to pulmonary disease. To do this we take the total number of pulmonary disease cases and divide that by the grand total (table 7.4).

This gives us a frequency for the occurrence of pulmonary disease. If exposure has nothing to do with pulmonary disease, then 0.25, or one-fourth, of the exposed population should have a health problem, and three-fourths should not. Since there are a total of 300 people in the exposed population (table 7.5), we would *expect* $300 \times 0.25 = 75$ of them to have the pulmonary disease and 300 –

Table 7.5   **Determining Expected Frequency of Disease in the Exposed Population**

Exposure	Pulmonary Disease Yes	Pulmonary Disease No	Row Total
Yes	90	210	**300**
No	85	315	400
Column total	175	525	700

Table 7.6   **Chi-Square Analysis of Data**

Exposure	Pulmonary Disease Yes	Pulmonary Disease No	Total
Yes	90 (75)[a]	210 (225)	300
No	85 (100)	315 (300)	400
Total	175	525	700

[a]Expected number of cases in parentheses.

75 = 225 not to have the disease. The same approach is used for the unexposed population with 400 × 0.25 = 100 expected to have the disease and 400 − 100 = 300 expected not to have the disease.

If you now go back to the original two-by-two table and put the expected numbers in parentheses in each appropriate box, you will be ready to begin the analysis of your data (table 7.6).

Mathematical Tables

You use chi-square by looking at the difference between the observed and expected values in each cell, performing a mathematical function on that difference, and adding up the results cell by cell to reach a total called a chi-square statistic. The logic of the chi-square is beyond the scope of this book; you can refer to the statistics section of a library to learn more about the procedure. The basic thrust of the test is to determine the difference between the observed number of people in a given cell (O) and the expected number of people for that cell (E): you then multiply that difference times itself, $(O–E) \times (O–E)$ or $(O–E)^2$, and divide that result by the value expected for that cell, $(O–E)^2/E$.

Table 7.7 Computation Table for Calculating Chi-Square

Exposure	Pulmonary Disease	O	E	O-E	$(O-E)^2$	$(O-E)^2/E$
Yes	Yes	90	75	15	225	3.00
Yes	No	210	225	15	225	1.00
No	Yes	85	100	15	225	2.25
No	No	315	300	15	225	0.75
Total						7.00

Note: O = observed; E = expected.

This is carried out for each cell, then these numbers are added together. A quick computation table keeps the math organized and allows you to progress at a pace that can be handled by any simple calculator (table 7.7).

Using the Chi-Square Statistic

The chi-square statistic in this example is 7.00. The problem is that this number in itself means very little. To make some sense out of this, you must go to the chi-square distribution table (table 7.8).

Before using the chi-square distribution table, there are a few things you need to know. The table is constructed around two items of information, the chi-square statistic, which you already have and know how to obtain, and a number called the degrees of freedom (df), which we will expand upon shortly; for now, this example has one degree of freedom.

The chi-square distribution table is entered along the row corresponding to the degrees of freedom your test has. Once you have the correct row, you read along that row looking for a number close to your chi-square statistic. For our example, the number for degrees of freedom (df) is one, so you use the first row in the body of the table and read along until you find a number close to 7.00, your chi-square statistic. From the table, 7.00 falls between 6.64 and 10.83. From here you read straight up to the column headings; 6.64 reads up to .01, and 10.83 yields the number .001. These two numbers are called *p*-values, and they are the standard to use in trying to determine if two groups are different.

P-Values

P-values are a statement about probability—specifically, the probability that the difference you observe is due solely to chance or

Table 7.8 Chi-Square Distribution Table

df	.99	.98	.95	.90	.80	.70	.50	.30	.20	.10	.05	.02	.01	.001
1	0.00016	0.00063	0.0039	0.016	0.064	0.15	0.46	1.07	1.64	2.71	3.84	5.41	6.64	10.83
2	0.02	0.04	0.10	0.21	0.45	0.71	1.39	2.41	3.22	4.60	5.99	7.82	9.21	13.82
3	0.12	0.18	0.35	0.58	1.00	1.42	2.37	3.66	4.64	6.25	7.82	9.84	11.34	16.27
4	0.30	0.43	0.71	1.06	1.65	2.20	3.36	4.88	5.99	7.78	9.49	11.67	13.28	18.46
5	0.55	0.75	1.14	1.61	2.34	3.00	4.35	6.06	7.29	9.24	11.07	13.39	15.09	20.52
6	0.87	1.13	1.64	2.20	3.07	3.83	5.35	7.23	8.56	10.64	12.59	15.03	16.81	22.46
7	1.24	1.56	2.17	2.83	3.82	4.67	6.35	8.38	9.80	12.02	14.07	16.62	18.48	24.32
8	1.65	2.03	2.73	3.49	4.59	5.53	7.34	9.52	11.03	13.36	15.51	18.17	20.09	26.12
9	2.09	2.53	3.32	4.17	5.38	6.39	8.34	10.66	12.24	14.68	16.92	19.68	21.67	27.88
10	2.56	3.06	3.94	4.86	6.18	7.27	9.34	11.78	13.44	15.99	18.31	21.16	23.21	39.59
11	3.05	3.61	4.58	5.58	6.99	8.15	10.34	12.90	14.63	17.28	19.68	22.62	24.72	31.26
12	3.57	4.18	5.23	6.30	7.81	9.03	11.34	14.01	15.81	18.55	21.03	24.05	26.22	32.91
13	4.11	4.76	5.89	7.04	8.63	9.93	12.34	15.12	16.98	19.81	22.36	25.47	27.69	34.53
14	4.66	5.37	6.57	7.79	9.47	10.82	13.34	16.22	18.15	21.06	23.68	26.87	29.14	36.12
15	5.23	5.98	7.26	8.55	10.31	11.72	14.34	17.32	19.31	22.31	25.00	28.26	30.58	37.70

Note: df = degrees of freedom.

natural variation and that your two groups are actually the same. Remember that probability ranges from zero to one, a probability of zero (.00) implying that something will never happen and a probability of one (1.00) implying that it will always happen. Another way to view p-values is to say they represent a measure of your belief that the two groups under study are actually the same. For the example, the p-value is somewhere between .01 and .001, or very close to .00. Therefore it is very unlikely that the two groups, exposed and unexposed, are the same with respect to the outcome of pulmonary disease.

The question arises of how small the p-value needs to be before you conclude that your two groups are different. This is a matter of debate in the scientific and statistical communities, with the "standard response" being that it should be equal to or less than .05. This reflects the conservative tendency of scientific professionals not to state that a difference exists unless there is a significant amount of evidence to support such a conclusion. However, since you are not out to establish indisputable evidence, but rather want to raise warning flags concerning potential health problems, if you get a p-value of less than .10 you should make note of that, and if the p-value is less than .02 you should seriously suspect that a difference (which implies a problem) exists between the two groups being studied.

Variations on the Two-by-Two Format

The example previously given is a good sample of the use of the chi-square analysis. However, in some situations you may have measured an outcome on a scale that is not simply an either/or combination (yes/no responses), but rather a range of responses, such as pulmonary problems requiring hospitalization, pulmonary problems requiring only prescription medication, and no evidence of pulmonary problems. The contributing factor being tested may also involve more than two alternatives, as when a stratified population has three or more "zones" (strata). The chi-square analysis can still be carried out on this type of material, in the same manner as before (table 7.9).

The computation table (table 7.10) is constructed as before, with the $(O-E)^2/E$ number generated for each cell and the result for each cell added to get the chi-square statistic. The only difference comes in using the chi-square distribution table—specifically, the degrees of freedom. As the dimensions of the original data table

Table 7.9   Chi-Square Example with an Exposure Gradient Divided into Three Zones and Two Levels of Symptoms

	Pulmonary Problem			
Zone	*Hospitalization Needed*	*Medication Needed*	*None*	*Total*
1	30 (24.3)	70 (51.4)	100 (124.3)	200
2	30 (30.4)	60 (64.3)	160 (155.4)	250
3	25 (30.4)	50 (64.3)	175 (155.4)	250
Totals	85	180	435	700

Note: The overall proportions for each of the health outcomes are:

Pulmonary disease
requiring hospitalization $85 \div 700 = 0.12$
Pulmonary disease
requiring prescription
medication $180 \div 700 = 0.26$
No evidence of pulmonary
disease $435 \div 700 = 0.62$

Table 7.10   Overall Proportions for Each of the Health Outcomes in Table 7.9

Pulmonary Problem	*O*	*E*	*O-E*	$(O-E)^2$	$(O-E)^2/E$
Zone 1					
Hospitalization needed	30	24.3	5.3	28.1	1.16
Medication needed	70	51.4	20.6	424.4	8.26
None	100	124.3	24.3	590.5	4.75
Zone 2					
Hospitalization needed	30	30.4	0.4	0.2	0.00
Medication needed	60	64.3	4.3	18.5	0.29
None	160	155.4	4.6	21.2	0.14
Zone 3					
Hospitalization needed	25	30.4	5.4	29.2	0.96
Medication needed	50	64.3	14.3	204.5	3.18
None	175	155.4	19.6	384.2	2.47
Total					21.21

Note: *O* = observed; *E* = expected.

change, so do the degrees of freedom. The new degrees of freedom can be obtained by adding up the number of rows (R) and columns (C), subtracting one from each, ($R-1$) and ($C-1$), then multiplying these two numbers ($R-1$) $\times$ ($C-1$). Therefore this example, which uses a three-by-three table, has ($3-1$) $\times$ ($3-1$) = 4 degrees of freedom. When you look along the row for four degrees of freedom to find a value near your chi-square statistic of 21.21, you run off the table. There is no number that large in the row for four degrees of freedom. You can conclude from this that the probability that the three zones have the pulmonary pattern they do simply by chance is less than .001 (the smallest p-value in the column heading on the far right). You must then strongly suspect that, whatever the difference is between the three zones, it is significantly affecting the development of pulmonary problems within each zone.

Comparing Your Population with Established Health Statistics

Occasionally, obtaining a comparison population is difficult, or there exist suitable local health statistics that make a comparison population unnecessary. In these cases you will compare the results from your study with reported standards for the health outcomes you are interested in. Since these health statistics are presented as rates of various sorts, one of the easiest ways to deal with your data is to generate a "reasonable bound" on the health statistic rate for a given health problem. Back to an example mentioned earlier: if the health statistics for a given disease showed a rate of ten per thousand, then in any population of one thousand people it would not be unexpected to see from four to sixteen cases of that disease, owing to normal variation within populations. Conversely, if you find sixteen cases of this disease in a population of one thousand people, even though your rate is sixteen per thousand you cannot say with reasonable certainty that your population is any different from a "normal population" that has a rate of ten per thousand. If this is confusing, a short test period of flipping a coin in series of ten tries, as described in chapter 4, should point out that, though the average number of heads you get when flipping the coin ten times is five, you actually see anywhere from two to eight heads in any given set of ten flips. In fact, in only about one-fourth of the sets of ten will you actually get five heads. The survey you have done is like a single series of ten flips. You may end up with exactly the published rate for some disease (just like getting five heads), you may get a number slightly different from the published rate (like seeing three or seven heads), or you may get a number that seems significantly different from the published rate (like getting all heads). Setting a "reasonable bound" on the estimate of the rate for a given health outcome lets you put a range around the published statistic so you can see if the observed rate for your population is within this bound. If your observed rate falls outside this range, then you must suspect that your population is different from the population used to generate the published health statistics. The possible advantages and pitfalls of using published health statistics have been discussed in previous chapters, and you should refresh your understanding of these if necessary. Unlike the chi-square analysis on two different populations, this technique, though it points out a potential problem, is weaker in its ability to suggest a possible cause.

The mathematical process for generating this "reasonable bound" is based on two factors: the "normal" rate for the health problem and the number of people in your population who could potentially develop that problem. The normal rate (P), in decimal notation, is multiplied by one minus that rate $(1-P)$ and divided by the number of susceptible people in your population (N), then the square root of this number is taken:

$$\sqrt{\frac{(P)\ (1-P)}{N}}.$$

This is considered the standard error of your estimate of a proportion (the rate of the disease). Most of the time (more than 90 percent) the estimate of the disease rate you get should fall within 1.65 times this standard error from the published rate:

$$1.65 \times \sqrt{\frac{(P)\ (1-P)}{N}}.$$

For example, with a published rate of 0.06 (six per hundred) and a population size of 1,000:

$$1.65 \times \sqrt{\frac{(.06)\ (1-.06)}{1,000}} = .0124.$$

Therefore, if the rate you observe is between 0.0476 and 0.0724,

$$.04 \longleftarrow \overset{\text{Range of Outcomes}}{\underset{\begin{array}{ccc} .0476 & .06 & .0724 \\ (.06-.0124) & & (.06+.0124) \end{array}}{\rule{0pt}{0pt}}} \longrightarrow .08 \qquad ,$$

or 48 and 72 per thousand, then you cannot say that your population is different from the "normal" population used to generate the health statistics. If your observed rate falls outside this reasonable bound, then you must take note of the situation, and if it falls well outside this range you should be concerned. In this case our range was 60 ± (plus or minus) 12 cases per thousand. If your observed rate is *outside* this range by more than half again the bound (12), that is, 0.5 × 12 = 6, this is a very important observation that suggests your population is significantly different from the normal population.

Since the calculations involved can be tedious and certain standard situations can be anticipated, table 7.11 has been generated to help you quickly estimate a reasonable bound for a few standard population sizes and rates. Remember that the population sizes down the left side represent the number of people you surveyed who could potentially develop a particular health problem, and the proportions across the top are the decimal representation of the normal rate as reported in published health statistics. The bounds used in this table are the same as those presented in the mathematical computation. Since you are generally interested in determining a directional difference, such as an *increase* in pulmonary disease or a *decrease* in number of births, the table gives a directional bound. Instead of using 1.65 times the standard error of the estimate (SEE), which gives a *bidirectional* measure and encompasses 90 percent of the expected outcomes, you use 1.28 times the SEE, which gives you a *one-directional* measure that encompasses 90 percent of the expected outcomes. If your actual population size or proportion for the health outcome does not appear in the table, you may do some sort of simple extrapolation by comparing your numbers with those that most closely bracket your data. Once again, these are ranges about a set proportion, and you still must solve the equation (background proportion + bound) or (background proportion – bound), where bound is equivalent to

$$1.28 \times \sqrt{\frac{(P)(1-P)}{N}} \, ,$$

which has been solved for you in this table. If your proportion (rate) falls near the edge of the reasonable bound, this constitutes a warning that the situation needs to be investigated further. If your proportion (rate) falls *outside* the bound by more than half again the size of the bound—that is, outside (background proportion ± 1.5 × bound)—then significant evidence exists to warrant special attention as to why your population is so different from the "normal" population. But keep in mind at all times the limitations of using published health statistics and realize that this evidence alone is not sufficient to attribute blame concerning the cause of the health problem; rather, it simply shows that the health problem is "real."

Other Statistical Considerations

Although the mathematical portions of statistics are fairly straightforward, a few aspects pertaining to experimental design and data interpretation need to be discussed. One factor, alluded to in the chapter on experimental design (chap. 4), is the concept of "power." The other factor is the role of "false positive" results in the analysis of data. We will briefly explain these concepts here so that you can appreciate the limits they can put on your study.

Power

With regard to a study and analysis, "power" means the ability to detect a difference between two populations given that the difference does exist. Although a number of things can contribute to a study's sensitivity (power), here we will deal only with three statistical factors: population, or more specifically sample size, natural variation, and the magnitude of the difference one is trying to detect. Since the equations needed to derive a measure of power are complicated, we will not get involved with them. Instead, table 7.12 presents a collection of possible study situations. With some orientation you should be able to use the table to help you design your study or to put your results in proper context.

The table is structured around two numbers: the background rate (proportion) for a given health effect is listed down the left side, and the relative increase over the background rate is across the top. The figures that constitute the body of the table are the number of people you would need to look at in both the exposed and the control populations in order to have an 80 percent chance of demonstrating that a difference does exist. For example, for a

The First Phase: Practical Guidelines

Table 7.11   Natural Variation around Published Proportions with a Variety of Population Sizes

Population Size	Expected Proportions from Published Health Statistics							
	.00001	.00002	.00004	.00008	.00016	.00032	.00064	.0013
50	.00057	.00081	.00114	.00162	.00229	.00324	.00548	.0065
100	.00040	.00057	.00081	.00114	.00162	.00229	.00324	.0046
150	.00030	.00047	.00066	.00093	.00132	.00187	.00264	.0037
200	.00029	.00040	.00057	.00081	.00114	.00162	.00229	.0032
250	.00026	.00036	.00051	.00072	.00102	.00145	.00205	.0029
300	.00023	.00033	.00047	.00066	.00093	.00132	.00187	.0026
350	.00022	.00031	.00043	.00061	.00087	.00122	.00173	.0024
400	.00020	.00029	.00040	.00057	.00081	.00114	.00162	.0023
450	.00019	.00027	.00038	.00054	.00076	.00108	.00153	.0022
500	.00018	.00026	.00036	.00051	.00072	.00102	.00145	.0020
600	.00017	.00023	.00033	.00047	.00066	.00093	.00132	.0019
700	.00015	.00022	.00031	.00043	.00061	.00087	.00122	.0017
800	.00014	.00020	.00029	.00040	.00057	.00081	.00114	.0016
900	.00013	.00019	.00027	.00038	.00054	.00076	.00108	.0015
1,000	.00013	.00018	.00026	.00036	.00051	.00072	.00102	.0014
1,200	.00012	.00017	.00023	.00033	.00047	.00066	.00093	.0013
1,400	.00011	.00015	.00022	.00031	.00043	.00061	.00087	.0012
1,600	.00010	.00014	.00020	.00029	.00040	.00057	.00081	.0011
1,800	.00010	.00013	.00019	.00027	.00038	.00054	.00076	.0011
2,000	.00009	.00013	.00018	.00026	.00036	.00051	.00072	.0010
2,500	.00008	.00011	.00016	.00023	.00032	.00046	.00065	.00091
3,000	.00007	.00010	.00015	.00021	.00030	.00042	.00059	.00094
3,500	.00007	.00010	.00014	.00019	.00027	.00039	.00055	.00077
4,000	.00006	.00009	.00013	.00018	.00026	.00036	.00051	.00072
4,500	.00006	.00009	.00012	.00017	.00024	.00034	.00048	.00068

health problem with a background rate of 0.02 (twenty per thousand), if you wanted to be able to detect a twofold increase (doubling) in your population, you would have to look at 874 people in your population and 874 people from a control population.

When we examine the table, two points become apparent. First, the larger the background rate for a given health problem, the smaller the study size needed to demonstrate a relative change in incidence. This results from the magnitude of the difference that accompanies "relative change." Second, as the severity of the difference changes (i.e., a twofold versus a fourfold increase), so does the number of people needed to demonstrate an effect. Table 7.13 represents the study size that will give you a 50 percent chance of demonstrating that something is going on.

These tables are important from both a pre- and a poststudy

Table 7.11 (continued)

Population Size	Expected Proportions from Published Health Statistics								
	.0026	.0051	.0102	.0205	.0410	.0819	.1638	.3277	.6554
50	.0091	.0129	.0182	.0256	.0359	.0496	.0670	.0850	.0860
100	.0065	.0091	.0129	.0181	.0254	.0351	.0474	.0601	.0608
150	.0053	.0075	.0105	.0148	.0207	.0287	.0387	.0491	.0497
200	.0046	.0065	.0091	.0128	.0179	.0248	.0335	.0425	.0430
250	.0041	.0058	.0081	.0115	.0160	.0222	.0300	.0380	.0385
300	.0037	.0053	.0074	.0105	.0146	.0203	.0274	.0347	.0351
350	.0035	.0049	.0069	.0097	.0136	.0188	.0253	.0321	.0325
400	.0032	.0046	.0064	.0091	.0127	.0176	.0237	.0300	.0304
450	.0030	.0043	.0061	.0085	.0120	.0165	.0223	.0283	.0287
500	.0029	.0041	.0058	.0081	.0113	.0157	.0212	.0269	.0272
600	.0026	.0037	.0053	.0074	.0104	.0143	.0193	.0245	.0248
700	.0024	.0035	.0049	.0069	.0096	.0133	.0179	.0227	.0230
800	.0023	.0032	.0046	.0064	.0090	.0124	.0168	.0212	.0215
900	.0022	.0030	.0043	.0060	.0085	.0117	.0158	.0200	.0203
1,000	.0020	.0029	.0041	.0057	.0080	.0111	.0150	.0190	.0192
1,200	.0019	.0026	.0037	.0052	.0073	.0101	.0137	.0173	.0176
1,400	.0017	.0024	.0034	.0048	.0068	.0094	.0127	.0161	.0163
1,600	.0016	.0023	.0032	.0045	.0063	.0088	.0118	.0150	.0152
1,800	.0015	.0022	.0030	.0043	.0060	.0083	.0112	.0142	.0143
2,000	.0014	.0020	.0029	.0041	.0057	.0078	.0106	.0134	.0136
2,500	.0013	.0018	.0026	.0036	.0051	.0070	.0095	.0120	.0122
3,000	.0012	.0017	.0024	.0033	.0046	.0064	.0086	.0110	.0111
3,500	.0011	.0015	.0022	.0031	.0043	.0059	.0080	.0102	.0103
4,000	.0010	.0014	.0020	.0029	.0040	.0056	.0075	.0095	.0096
4,500	.00096	.0014	.0019	.0027	.0038	.0052	.0071	.0090	.0091

perspective. For prestudy purposes, if you know the background rate for the particular health problem that interests you and have in mind the type of increase you would like to be able to detect in your population (say a twofold increase, or doubling over normal), then tables 7.12 and 7.13 will tell you the size of the study necessary to have an 80 percent or a 50 percent chance of demonstrating such an effect. Therefore you can plan the size of your study to give yourself the degree of power you want. Increasing the number of people in your study will always increase your power. These tables can also help you realize the limitations of your study. For studies involving rare health conditions you must study a large number of people to have even a small chance of seeing sizable increases over background rates. In this situation you must either accept this potential problem and continue with

Table 7.12 Population Sizes for Exposed and Control Groups Needed to Have an 80 Percent Chance of Demonstrating a Significant Difference between Two Populations

Background Rate	Relative Increase over Background Rate							
	2	4	6	8	10	12	14	16
.00001	1,900,00	345,000	170,000	110,000	83,853	66,338	54,802	46,650
.00002	930,000	170,000	86,444	56,703	41,923	33,165	27,398	23,322
.00004	460,000	85,755	43,217	28,347	20,958	16,579	13,695	11,657
.00008	230,000	42,872	21,604	14,170	10,475	8,286	6,844	5,825
.00016	120,000	21,430	10,798	7,081	5,234	4,139	3,418	2,909
.00032	57,862	10,709	5,394	3,536	2,613	2,066	1,706	1,451
.00064	28,915	5,349	2,693	1,764	1,303	1,029	850	722
.00128	14,442	2,669	1,342	878	648	511	421	358
.00256	7,206	1,328	667	435	320	252	207	176
.005	3,587	659	329	214	157	123	100	85
.01	1,778	324	160	103	75	58	47	39
.02	874	156	76	48	34	25	20	16
.04	422	73	34	20	13	9	7	5
.05	340	57	26	15	10	6	4	3
.10	155	23	9	4	1			
.15	93	12	3					
.20	62	6						
.25	44	3						
.30	31							
.35	23							
.40	16							
.45	11							
.50	7							

Table 7.13 Population Sizes for Exposed and Control Groups Needed to Have a 50 Percent Chance of Demonstrating a Significant Difference between Two Populations

Background Rate	*Relative Increase over Background Rate*							
	2	4	6	8	10	12	14	16
.00001	810,000	150,000	75,765	49,699	36,745	29,070	24,015	20,442
.00002	410,000	75,162	37,880	28,848	18,371	14,533	12,006	10,220
.00004	200,000	37,579	18,938	12,422	9,184	7,265	6,001	5,108
.00008	100,000	18,787	9,467	6,209	4,590	3,631	2,999	2,553
.00016	50,724	9,391	4,732	3,103	2,293	1,814	1,498	1,275
.00032	25,355	4,693	2,364	1,550	1,145	906	748	636
.00064	12,671	2,344	1,180	773	571	451	373	317
.00128	6,329	1,169	588	385	284	224	185	157
.00256	3,158	583	292	191	141	111	91	77
.005	1,572	289	144	94	69	54	44	37
.01	780	142	70	45	33	26	21	17
.02	383	69	33	21	15	11	9	7
.04	185	32	15	9	6	4	3	2
.05	149	25	12	7	4	3	2	1
.10	68	10	4	2	1			
.15	41	5	2					
.20	28	3						
.25	19	1						
.30	14							
.35	10							
.40	7							
.45	5							
.50	3							

the study, remembering that you *don't actually know* how great the effect is in your community, or eliminate this section of your study, which unfortunately doesn't help anyone. You may easily find yourself working on something with little hope of success. Seriously evaluate the process beforehand so as to appreciate the work that lies ahead. If, after the fact, you are unable to demonstrate a health problem in your community, remind yourself of the power of your study. Also remember that it is not uncommon for studies with very little power to be conducted and that just because you could not demonstrate a difference between your population and some "normal" population does not necessarily mean no problem exists.

Last, if you partition your population into subpopulations based on contributing factors such as smoking history, age, or sex, some of the sensitivity gained from focusing on more susceptible subgroups may in part be offset by a drop in power. Don't go too far in delineating highly specific subgroups of your population.

False Positives

A "false positive" occurs when a difference appears to exist between two populations, or between the study population and some standard proportion, when in fact there is no real difference at all. This goes back to the role of natural variation and the fact that we must use some standard for decision making. As discussed earlier, scientists use a p-value of .05 to determine whether their results are significant. This means that up to 5 percent of the times when they make that decision they will be wrong. This is because it is so difficult to *prove* certain types of material; sometimes you can do no more than collect a significant amount of evidence. The scientific community has come to accept this false-positive rate as an appropriate trade-off between making an incorrect decision (false positive) when no difference exists and doing so when in fact a difference does exist (false negative).

With the statistical methods given in this chapter, a false positive rate of one in ten (10 percent) has been accepted. This means that about 10 percent of your comparisons will come out as possibly significant. Therefore, that one or two indicators of health show increased levels compared with some "normal" group does not necessarily mean that a real difference, or problem, exists. Once again this is a trade-off. Ideally you want no false positives, yet you need some standard so you can at least begin to identify possible health problems. As we mentioned in discussing chi-square and reasonable bounds, a p-value of about .10 constitutes a warning that you should look further. With a p-value of less than .02, or if the "reasonable bound" is more than one and one-half times the bound width away from the normal rate, then a significant amount of evidence exists that a problem (the observed difference in health status between two populations) is real. You need temperance and understanding when analyzing your data. Any comparison that shows a warning flag (p-value of .10 or less) should be looked at further to determine if specific subpopulations exist that are experiencing the bulk of the increase in adverse health conditions.

Part 3

The Second Phase
Assistance, Causality, and Legal Implications

8   Where Do You Go from Here?
Assistance from State and Federal Agencies, Confirmation of the Problem, and Analytical Epidemiology

Ellen K. Silbergeld

After you have prepared your report using the methods presented in the previous chapter, several things can happen. If you have concluded that a health problem exists, your community group or task force can meet with local officials to assess various alternatives. The state and federal officials responsible for protecting your health should also be notified. Your first job will be convincing the person or agency you approach that your results are accurate; a well-prepared report will greatly aid you at this point. Once everyone agrees that a problem exists, the next step is to negotiate for professional studies to confirm the problem, for chemical analyses to identify causative agents, for a mechanism to stop exposure and prevent it in the future, and for some means of treating present or future adverse health effects. Of course this is easier said than done, and you will undoubtedly meet resistance from officials while you are also under pressure from your community to get results. In a sense the health survey is a tool that will get you about halfway to your ultimate goals, and for many communities the obstacles are never overcome.

Now that it is clear where the health survey fits into the overall process, you can move from the thinking phase to the doing phase.

165

After you complete an investigation of health effects in your community, you will be faced with choices for action. Here we assume that you decide something more must be done. This may include obtaining further information on health, getting the source of toxic chemicals cleaned up, or obtaining compensation for damage to property or health. First, and most important, remember your commitments to your friends and neighbors and arrange for a full presentation of study results to all who are potentially affected. Remember to deal sensitively and discreetly with everyone involved.

Your choices are obviously influenced by the outcome of the study. In all cases, successful mobilization of resources to attain your goals ultimately depends upon the effectiveness of your organization and your persistence in political action.

Obtaining Further Information

After completing your health study, you may want to enlist the assistance of organizations or people with greater resources, more access to medical information, and medical or clinical skills and facilities. Citizens in Triana, Alabama, and in Michigan involved the Centers of Disease Control in extensive and long-term health studies of DDT and PCBs.

It is important to realize that as soon as others are involved in further health studies in your community, control and direction pass out of your hands. Their goals and objectives may not be the same as yours, since in many cases they need to satisfy the more exacting criteria of scientific research, and they may be affected by economic and political pressures. It usually takes such organizations a relatively long time to get their further studies under way, in part because they must submit any projects to clinical research committees or other forms of review, and in part because they have to coordinate people or departments within their institutions.

Your relations with such outside investigators will be most succesful if you keep in mind that both sides have gains and losses in working together. You retain the ultimate power of not agreeing to participate—a powerful weapon in negotiating an acceptable and comprehensive study, because the research can be irreparably damaged if large numbers of people decline to take part. On their side, they have the power to determine the scope of the study, the types of questions to be answered, and the methods of data analysis. You can and should demand to take as active a role as possible in the analysis of the study, but you should respect their need to conduct it independently. The value of their work will largely depend upon others' perception of its objectivity and independence. Before you agree to participate, make sure the goals of the study are acceptable to you and that you are satisfied with schedules, procedures, access to information, and the like.

Further studies may be necessary to resolve important issues of concern to your community or to provide various types of information on health effects, such as biopsies to determine individual exposure more precisely. Three types of resources are available for assistance in conducting further research: private medical services (including hospitals, health maintenance organizations, and private physicians); universities, schools of public health, and medical schools; and public health departments in the local, county, state, and federal levels.

Private medical services can get interested in conducting community health studies, particularly if they are involved in preventive health care and, most important, if they are responsible for the medical expenses of many people in the community. For example, the Kaiser Permanente health care organization in Santa Clara county, California, has taken part in studying whether there has been an increase in birth defects associated with exposure to 1,1,1-trichloroethane in drinking water.

Universities, schools of public health, and medical schools, particularly those with departments of community medicine or epidemiology, are often very interested in conducting intensive studies of community health. Among the schools of public health and medical schools that have already been involved in such studies are those of the State University of New York at Binghamton, Johns Hopkins University, Harvard, Boston University, the University of Massachusetts, the University of California at Los Angeles, and the University of Texas.

Public health agencies include local public health offices, county and state agencies, and the federal Public Health Service (Centers for Disease Control [CDC]). These organizations are set up by law and funded by taxes specifically to protect public health and investigate potential causes of community illness. Often they can bring to their work extensive resources, personnel, and experience.

It is difficult to recommend a particular source for obtaining assistance with further health studies. Unfortunately, all organizations can be hampered by political and other pressures, and every organization is constrained by the funds available. You need to investigate work the group has done on similar topics, which you do get by requesting copies of publications describing their research. Keep in mind that every study of your community in a sense reduces the probability of further studies, so that as far as possible you need to ensure that the best possible study is done on this second round.

If you cannot get a local public health official to help you, you can call the CDC directly; follow up your telephone call with a letter describing your community, the results of your own study, and your judgment as to the source and types of toxic exposure. Send a copy of your correspondence to your representative in Congress; if you do not get a response from government agencies, you can ask her or him to intervene. Concern for health transcends politics: the citizens of Fort Smith, Arkansas, used this process to file a request for action (from the Environmental Protection Agency) through Congressman John Hammerschmidt, a conservative Republican.

It is always useful to notify the federal Public Health Service of your study, because they maintain data banks on health and potential dangers to health. Even if you get no initial action from this source, your request may be acted on later (for example, if other similar results are observed or there is a chemical fire at a dumpsite). Moreover, your letter serves as official notification of your study and your concerns, which may be useful in the future.

Getting a Cleanup

One of the main reasons for communities to undertake health studies is the existence of an obvious source of chemical exposure, such as a hazardous waste dump. Even if your health study does not conclusively show adverse health effects in your community, you may still be concerned about getting the dump site cleaned up. To accomplish this you have several resources. The principal one is a federal law, the Comprehensive Rehabilitation and Environmental Compensation and Liability Act of 1980 (CERCLA), better known as Superfund.

Your state may have, and certainly should have, its own "Superfund" law to finance the state's share of the federal program and to provide for dump sites not covered by the federal cleanup (such as sites with lower priority in the national ranking system).

Superfund provides the EPA with the authority and the funding to identify such dump sites, develop action plans, and clean up the waste. Unfortunately, as with anything else, it takes persistence and political organization to get Superfund to work in your community. The Environmental Defense Fund (EDF) has just published a citizens' guide to Superfund (available from the Toxic Chemicals Program of EDF, 1525 18th Street NW, Washington, D.C. 20036) to help you get Superfund to work effectively in your community.

As a federal program, Superfund can be difficult to activate. Many states now also have their own Superfund programs, designed to provide for dump site cleanups. You need to consult your state department of environmental protection or natural resources to find out the details of such programs and how to activate them. If your state government offices are not helpful, an inquiry through a state representative may be more effective.

The Public Health Service has new resources provided through Superfund specifically to conduct health studies and to set up long-term health registries of people likely to have been exposed to toxic chemicals from hazardous waste dump sites. It took a lawsuit by EDF to accomplish this, but the EPA will soon be forced to release millions of dollars for these purposes. Table 8.1 lists the regional offices of the EPA.

Compensation

If in the course of your study you establish that you or others may have suffered specific health damage or that your property has depreciated as a result of exposure to toxic substances, you have the right to seek compensation.

From a scientific medical point of view, we should make the following points. Legal suits are strongest under these three conditions:

- Fairly serious health effects have occurred (children born with birth defects, persons developing liver disease, for example).
- Chemical exposure has been directly measured in people or in their food or drinking water.
- The chemicals detected are already well defined and, ideally, already regulated or banned as toxic.

In situations where potential health effects—such as increased *risk* of cancer—are alleged, or where toxic substances have not yet been measured directly in people or are a complex mixture not yet fully investigated, it will be more difficult to build a case, but this has successfully been done in at least one instance.

At present the federal Superfund law does not provide for this

Table 8.1   Regional Offices of the Environmental Protection Agency

Region	States Covered	Address
1	CT, MA, ME, NH, RI, VT	John F. Kennedy Federal Building Room 2203 Boston, MA 02203
2	NJ, PR, VI, NY	26 Federal Plaza Room 1009 New York, NY 10007
3	MD, PA, VA, WV, DE, DC	Curtis Building 6th and Walnut Streets Philadelphia, PA 19106
4	AL, FL, GA, KY, MS, NC, SC, TN	345 Courtland Street NE Atlanta, GA 30308
5	IL, IN, MI, MN, OH, WI	230 Dearborn Street Chicago, IL 60604
6	AR, LA, NM, TX	First International Building 1201 Elm Street Dallas, TX 75270
7	IA, KS, MO, NE	324 East 11th Street Kansas City, MO 64106
8	CO, MT, ND, SD, UT, WY	1860 Lincoln Street Denver, CO 80203
9	AS, AZ, CA, GU, HI; NV, TT of US, Cmw. Mariannas	215 Fremont Street San Francisco, CA 94105
10	AK, ID, OR, WA	1200 6th Avenue Seattle, WA 98101

Dr. E. B. Houck, Director
Center for Environmental Health
Centers for Disease Control
Atlanta, Georgia 30333

type of compensation (known as victim compensation), though it does contain provisions covering damage to natural resources and the environment. There is considerable interest in Congress in expanding Superfund or creating a new law to address the issue of compensation for damage to health by dump site exposure.

What communities have sought compensation for chemical exposure? In Kellogg, Idaho, parents sued a smelter company (Gulf and Western) for dumping so much lead in their community that their children were severely poisoned. Several of these cases have been settled out of court. Citizens in Triana, Alabama, have won cases against Olin for dumping DDT in their community and contaminating their food supply. In San Jose, California, families have sued Fairchild Industries for contaminating their drinking water with trichloroethane, holding that several of their children's birth defects were associated with this exposure. There are many citizens' suits against Hooker Chemical Company in Hyde Park and Niagara Falls, New York.

To determine the advisability of bringing a legal suit for compensation and to judge the strength of your case, you need legal counsel. In addition, there is an organization of lawyers who have specialized in this area of law and can be consulted by citizens—the Trial Lawyers for Public Justice (2000 P Street, NW, Washington, D.C. 20036, tel. [202]463-8600).

Next

There is more to do. Chemical contamination of the environment has only recently been recognized as one of the most important concerns of our modern life, in large part as a result of citizens' urgent concern about their communities and their health. Action continues to depend upon the focused political expression of that concern.

We need action on two levels. First, we must work more quickly and comprehensively to correct the problems caused by past mismanagement. At Price's landfill in New Jersey, trichloroethylene, lead, benzene, and other toxic chemicals are moving through the ground toward the drinking water supply of Atlantic City. The EPA has stockpiled activated carbon to place in municipal water systems in an attempt to remove these chemicals once they reach the acquifer. In Dade County, Florida, chemicals escaping from the 58th Street landfill have already contaminated several well fields that provide drinking water for Hialeah Gardens and the suburbs of Miami. The wells have been shut down, but the chemical front continues to move.

These are admissions of failure—policies of retreat. Relying on these policies, we shall slowly or quickly surrender more and more of our country and its resources to an irreversible state of chemically induced degradation and loss.

Your community knows firsthand what this really means. You know it is not possible to move away soon enough, to close down wells fast enough. What can you do?

- If your state has no Superfund law, work to get one written, proposed, and passed by your state legislature.
- If you have identified a source of chemical contamination, work to get it corrected—through federal and state Superfund programs, or through state and federal laws on pollution control if it is an active source.

The other important direction for your efforts is the future. We must prevent the conditions that permit chemical contamination to occur. This means more than keeping industries or disposal facilities out of your community because of their *potential* to pollute the environment. There are laws and regulations that can effectively prevent dangerous or incompetent operation of such sources. You can:

- Attend local and state National Pollution Discharge System (NPDES) discharge permit hearings and be actively informed about the conditions under which industries operate in your community. Citizens in Michigan have been very effective at overseeing the way Dow Chemical Company will be permitted to discharge its wastes.
- Demand public hearings for any new hazardous waste dump, at which the industry or waste disposal company must present details on its operations that might affect your community. Citizens in Calcasieu, Louisiana, and in South Baltimore, Maryland, have used this process to get a great deal of information on the intentions of waste disposal managers in their communities.
- Join local and national networks to effectively inform Congress of your support for strong laws to regulate environmental protection and handling—the Clean Air Act, Clean Water Act, Resource Conservation and Recycling Act, and Toxic Substances Control Act all require periodic reauthorization. Widespread citizen pressure will save these laws from being weakened or restricted.

9 What Kind of Evidence Do You Need?
Legal Implications of Acute and Chronic Effects

William E. Townsley

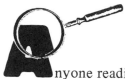

nyone reading this handbook has probably asked:

- Why are my neighbors and I being forced to defend ouselves against a toxic assault taking place in our own homes, schools, churches, parks, and public streets?
- Why haven't public health authorities been given the responsibility and the resources to protect us?
- Why has the public given the toxic waste generator a major role in ascertaining the harm from its toxic waste? Isn't it rather foolish to assign this responsibility to a party with such an obvious conflict of interest?
- Do victims of toxic harm have any legal rights?
- What can we, the public, do to better protect ourselves?

As we discuss issues raised by these questions, you will better understand why effective protection depends upon adequate identification of toxic harm, its victims, and its causes.

As more and more information accumulates on the role a toxic agent plays in causing harm, such a causal role may progress from mere speculation to distinct possibility, onward to probability, and at times even to scientific certainty. The facts necessary to build a reliable bridge between speculation and certainty are often

173

available only to the toxic waste generator (TWG). Therefore the TWG can prevent, stall, or weaken this evidentiary bridge by neglecting to compile necessary data, for example, exposure information, and by withholding proprietary data needed by health investigators, for example, information needed for epidemiologic studies.[1]

The TWG, in its adversary relationship with the public, has often promoted ignorance and uncertainty as to the identity of toxic harm, its victims, and its causes. The resulting ignorance and uncertainty have been effectively used to thwart public regulation of the TWG and enable it to evade its responsibility to toxic harm victims.

In this chapter we will discuss a hypothetical toxic harm claim so as to illustrate some of the complex legal and factual considerations involved. Our hypothetical claim will involve a victim, exposed both inside and outside the workplace, who has chronic disease (cancer) allegedly caused by contamination of the ambient air by neighborhood industries over a long period of time.

We should keep in mind that toxic harm victims, both inside and outside the workplace, have fared poorly in obtaining legal relief. Occupational disease kills over 100,000 workers every year, and three or four times that many are disabled. Yet only 5 percent of occupational disease victims are compensated, and for that 5 percent the compensation is little and late.

While cancer is the toxic harm in our hypothetical claim, we should recognize that cancer may not prove to be the most serious type of damage. We know that there is also reproductive, teratogenic, and behavioral harm, but we have no idea of the magnitude and, unfortunately, too little is being done to understand the nature and proportion of such harm. After reviewing this hypothetical claim, I will further analyze how and why the public has found itself unprotected in dealing with toxic harm. Then I will offer a relatively simple plan as a partial solution.

In this chapter I have given few references, since the material is not written for the legal community and scientific material has

---

1. Throughout this chapter I will express a number of views and conclusions based on my personal involvement in chronic disease litigation in which many of the nation's leading petrochemical companies gave testimony and other evidence of their activities in ascertaining the cancer dangers arising out of their operations. The industry evidence touched on the companies' limited contribution to exposure data, carcinogenicity research, and epidemiologic studies.

been adequately discussed and referenced in other chapters. Moreover, my own views and conclusions have been strongly influenced by knowledge and experience gained from personal involvement in cancer litigation.

Duty of the Toxic Waste Generator to Ascertain Dangers

A toxic waste generator (TWG) has a legal duty to ascertain the dangers arising out of its operations, including the disposal of its toxic waste into the atmosphere, into the waterways, and on and into the earth.[2] The TWG can perform this legal duty (1) by identifying, measuring, and recording the exposure creating possible risks; (2) by conducting appropriate toxicity studies; (3) by conducting well-designed epidemiologic studies of populations at risk; (4) by developing and using effective methods of biological monitoring; and (5) by keeping abreast of pertinent medical and scientific literature and new developments.

Unfortunately the TWGs, for the most part, have ignored their legal duty to discover the dangers created by their toxic waste. For example, the great majority of commercial chemicals have never been tested for risk of causing chronic disease and reproductive harm. The TWGs have failed to conduct adequate epidemiologic studies of their employees, even in respect to workplace exposure to confirmed animal carcinogens. This breach of duty has prevented an adequate identification of toxic harm, its victims, and its causes. Instead of being punished for their duty breach, the TWGs have been rewarded in at least two respects: in avoiding the expense of performing their duty, and in escaping virtually all responsibility to their toxic harm victims.

Statement of a Hypothetical Claim

Jim Brewster, age thirty-two, has recently been told by his physician that he has brain cancer—a type identified as glioblastoma multiforme. The prognosis is poor.

At age five, Jim moved to Jackson, Texas, and his father went to work for Able Chemical Company's large petrochemical complex there. After Jim graduated from Jackson High School, he too went to work for Able Chemical and is now assistant operator of a unit

---

2. See *Borel v. Fibreboard Paper Products Corp.*, 403 F. 2d 1076 (5th cir. 1973), holding a duty of a manufacturer to test for dangers and to keep abreast of medical and scientific literature.

that makes ethyl benzene. Other units at Able make benzene, styrene, vinyl chloride, and polyvinyl chloride.

From age five until he was about fourteen, Jim lived about one mile northwest of Able Chemical. His other two residences have been two and three miles from Able. Adjoining Able is Baker Chemical Company, the other substantial petrochemical complex in Jackson that also produces the products named above. Jim's residences have been approximately the same distance from Baker as from Able.

Jim is aware that a recent epidemiologic study of Able workers by a government agency revealed an incidence of brain cancer significantly above that in the general population. Also, another epidemiologic study of a similar but distant petrochemical plant showed a significant excess of brain cancer. Both Able Chemical and the distant company did their own epidemiologic studies and reached a contrary conclusion, finding that no such excess existed.

Jim talked to a lawyer who had recently won a workers' compensation case for the widow of an Able Chemical worker who died from brain cancer. After the lawyer reviewed the pertinent data and records, he told Jim that he had a good chance of winning a workers' compensation claim and perhaps even a fair chance on a traditional suit against Able and Baker jointly.

Jim's lawyer saw a chance to prove that a contributing cause to Jim's brain cancer was his exposure, both inside and outside the workplace, to the carcinogenic waste of Able and Baker, which contaminated the ambient air.

With this simplified version of the facts, let's examine some of the evidence problems and some pertinent principles to be applied to the facts.

Reconstructing Past Toxic Exposure

Jim's lawyer will aid a group of scientists (industrial hygienists, inhalation toxicologists, industrial chemists, meteorologists, and so on), who are experts in estimating toxic exposures, in the difficult and expensive task of reconstructing, as evidence permits, the toxic exposure from both Able Chemical and Baker Chemical to which Jim was subjected from 1955 (when he moved to Jackson) until his brain cancer was diagnosed in 1982.

Based on experience, Jim's lawyer is not surprised to learn that very little air sampling and analysis for specific compounds has ever been performed in Jackson, and that the few exposure data available are virtually useless. Likewise, the air monitoring data within the Able and Baker facilities have been found grossly inadequate.

If the emissions data were reasonably accurate during the disease latency and exposure period (twenty-seven years), and if necessary meterological data were available, Jim's primary exposure expert might undertake atmospheric modeling in an effort to scientifically quantify past exposures. While such modeling may be too difficult and expensive in most cases, expert evidence on the atmospheric transport of industrial pollutants will help explain the disease risk to populations outside the workplace.

The attorney, through court procedures, will obtain from Able Chemical (and also Baker Chemical) a plot plan of the Jackson plant(s) showing various process units, storage facilities, shipping locations, and all emission points; a pertinent history on each process unit since 1955; pertinent material balances; emissions inventories filed with the Texas Air Control Board; air emissions data furnished to federal agencies; and all air monitoring records on select compounds.

The exposure expert will review any government studies (by EPA, OSHA, NIOSH, or state and local regulatory agencies) of emissions from the plants of Able and Baker and from other plants with similar process units.

Some toxic substances have known odor thresholds and have such distinct odors that many workers can recognize their presence. These workers may testify about the existence and frequency of such detectable odors in the areas where Jim lived and moved about.

Jim's attorney will be able to make a broad estimate of the carcinogenic waste of Able and Baker that contaminated the ambient air where Jim lived and worked. Such an estimate may include total hydrocarbons as well as select compounds that are known or likely carcinogens. The exposure data, once compiled, must be reviewed by Jim's cancer causation expert, who will determine whether they are adequate, when considered together with epidemiologic, toxicologic, and other data, to prove (more likely than not) that such exposure was a contributing, legal cause of Jim's brain tumor.

Able and Baker may complain about the imprecision of the reconstructed exposure data, but such complaints should fall on deaf ears. After all, they had a duty to ascertain the dangers arising out of their operations, and had they performed such duty they necessarily would have compiled the exposure data, which would then have been available (by subpoena) to the toxic harm victims. In other words, after breaching its duty to compile such exposure data, a TWG should not be heard to complain about the quality of the reconstructed data. In the interest of justice, the court should appoint a master to reconstruct the exposure data at the expense of the derelict TWG. The master (master in chancery) is a judicial officer appointed by courts of equity to hear testimony and make reports that, when approved by the presiding judge, become the decision of the court.

We will assume that the exposure data have been reconstructed, that the court has found the methods satisfactory, and that the data have been admitted into evidence.

Proving Legal Causation

Jim will be required to prove that his exposure to the toxic waste of Baker Chemical (while outside the workplace) and Able Chemical (both inside Able and outside) was a legal cause of his brain tumor. Other facts must also be established, but proving legal causation is a major hurdle for the toxic harm victim. Under some legal theories (e.g., strict liability) the claimant must prove only that the exposure in question was a "producing cause," while under other legal theories (e.g., negligence) proving "proximate cause" will be required.

There may be several legal causes of an event or condition (such as toxic harm). To prove "producing cause" some jurisdictions require only proof of "cause-in-fact," which means the harm would not have occurred at the time it did but for the exposure in question; other jurisdictions require proof that the cause was a "substantial factor" in bringing about such harm; and still others require both cause-in-fact and substantial factor evidence.

To prove "proximate cause," the claimant, in addition to proving producing cause, must also show that the TWG should have foreseen that the same or similar harm might reasonably have occurred because of such exposure. Some jurisdictions will permit the claimant to lump the combined effect of the toxic exposures of the various TWG defendants and then prove (more likely than not) that such combined effect was a legal cause of the harm, leaving it to each defendant to separate, if it can, its contribution, if any, to the total toxic harm. However, other jurisdictions will still require the claimant to prove the contribution of each TWG defendant to the total harm.

Jim must present expert opinion evidence that his toxic exposure from Able and Baker caused his brain tumor. The expert may acknowledge that several factors probably contributed to Jim's cancer and may be of the opinion that one of those factors was Jim's exposure to the toxic waste of Able and Baker that contaminated the ambient air. Of course no one can say with absolute certainty what caused Jim's brain tumor, and the law does not require such certainty. Jim must only prove (through his expert) that the toxic exposure was more likely than not a contributing, legal cause.

Epidemiologic Studies

While not necessarily the best, epidemiologic studies are the most understandable evidence of cancer causation by toxic exposures. These studies have been described in earlier chapters. Epidemiologic studies may link a certain type of cancer with a certain compound (e.g., leukemia with benzene), or with a certain industry (e.g., brain cancer with the petrochemical industry), or with a certain occupation (e.g., respiratory cancer with pipefitting).

The design of an epidemiologic study is critical and vitally affects validity. For any epidemiologic study to merit serious consideration in a legal setting, it should be made available for peer review, that is, be subject to critical review by other epidemiologists.

The strength of a positive epidemiologic study is expressed in statistical terms. Scientific significance (high degree of certainty) and legal significance (more likely than not) are not the same thing. A nonpositive epidemiologic study should not be regarded as evidence that no risk exists, but rather should be considered as failing to establish a risk. The courts are beginning to accept (as they should) positive epidemiologic studies as supporting an inference of a causal connection between exposure and toxic harm. The TWG can be expected to oppose such use of statistical evidence when unfavorable, since it may make the TWG responsible to its toxic harm victims. The TWG, of course, wants to avoid this responsibility and can successfully do so as long as the victims are denied sufficient causation evidence.

Jim's causation expert, as a basis for his professional opinion, may rely upon several types of evidence, one being government epidemiologic studies showing a significant excess of brain cancer among petrochemical workers. The expert for Able and Baker will be critical of the government studies and will seek to use the industry-sponsored epidemiologic studies to rebut causation. The industry-sponsored studies will lack credibility if their design is poor or if their data have not been made available for peer review. Jim's expert may strengthen his opinion with epidemiologic studies not involving the petrochemical industry or the implicated compounds. An example would be studies showing that neighborhood populations are subjected to the same risks (though to a lesser degree as distance increases) as the workers within a given plant.

The court (judge) will determine whether the causation expert can use such epidemiologic studies in arriving at his opinion. The jury, by contrast, will determine the weight to be given any such study. The jury can accept a study's findings as factual, reject the study in toto, or accept some parts and reject others. Such evaluation will be reflected in the weight the jury gives to the opinion of the causation expert.

Toxicity Studies

Toxicity studies may be relevant in proving that the carcinogenic waste of Able and Baker was a legal cause of Jim's brain cancer. Significantly, our nation makes major public health decisions based on the results of animal studies. This shows our high degree of confidence in the validity of extrapolation from animals to man. In our hypothetical case, Jim's causation expert may use toxicity studies, along with other evidence, to strengthen his opinion on the causal link between Jim's brain tumor and his toxic exposure to the chemical waste of Able and Baker. In some instances a causation expert would be justified in relying upon toxicity studies alone to support an opinion of legal causation. An example would be where an animal carcinogen is very potent, the cancer victim has a history of substantial exposure to that particular carcinogen, the victim's cancer is similar (organ and type) to that induced by the carcinogen in animal species, and the type of cancer is not common.

Epidemiologic studies remain the evidence of choice for those who demand a victim body count before accepting positive animal studies. However, well designed two-year animal studies may prove to have greater overall validity than epidemiologic studies. The uncertainty in extrapolation is arguably smaller than the uncertainty from confounding factors of uncontrolled conditions that beset even the better epidemiologic studies. Where animal studies of a chemical prove to be nonpositive, the TWG may argue that such studies are valid evidence of the safety of the substance. However, when such studies prove positive, the TWG will be critical of extrapolation, both as to species and as to dosage. Again we see the TWG, in an adversary relationship with the public, seeking to place the burden of uncertainty on its potential victims.

Toxicity studies, standing alone, may or may not support an opinion of legal causation in Jim's case. In any event, such studies will give added strength to an opinion on causation. Toxicity data will show that certain compounds in the toxic waste of Able and Baker have an affinity for the brain. Moreover, one of the compounds (vinyl chloride monomer) is a potent animal (and human) carcinogen, with the brain as one of the target organs. Also, styrene would be suspected of making a contribution because of its similarity to vinyl chloride in chemical structure and because styrene (or its metabolites) is a likely carcinogen and/or promotor.

Jim's causation expert may not wish to isolate vinyl chloride as a legal cause but may prefer to implicate the total chemical emissions, which contain not only known and suspected carcinogens, but also a number of untested (or inadequately tested) compounds. The expert can correctly point out that, while vinyl chloride monomer is very likely a causal factor, there are still other carcinogens and promoters in such toxic waste that will likewise make their contribution to Jim's brain tumor.

Structure-Activity Data

The causation expert, with his background in toxicology, knows that the great majority of chemical compounds found in the environment have never been tested for carcinogenicity. This failure to test has created a need to predict, as scientifically as possible, the toxic effects of untested chemicals. This need has been partially met by studying the reactivity of untested compounds with DNA and by classifying the various chemicals according to their molecular structure. These predictive tools cannot support a conclusion that a given chemical is or is not a carcinogen, but such characteristics can be considered when evaluating toxicity and epidemiologic studies.

The Role of Principles of Carcinogenesis
in Legal Causation

All doses of carcinogens, no matter how small, are likely to contribute to the total carcinogenic effect. Jim's expert may point out that the effect of multiple carcinogens is at least additive, and in some instances is synergistic. This means that Jim's exposure to vinyl chloride, benzene, and other carcinogens in the toxic waste of Able and Baker had a causal role in his brain tumor. Moreover, there may have been noncarcinogenic substances present that played a causal role as cancer promoters. Keep in mind that most, if not all, carcinogens are also cancer promoters. However, not all promoters are carcinogens.

The intensity and duration of the dosage of carcinogens affects the latency period of cancer—the time between initial exposure and tumor formation. The greater the cumulative dosage of carcinogens, the shorter the latency period; and of course a reduced dosage will extend the latency period. Proving legal causation is made easier by the well-accepted principle of carcinogenesis that dosage directly affects the cancer latency period. By this principle, Jim's expert can state with confidence that Jim's brain tumor would not have appeared *when it did* except for his toxic exposure. In other words, without the exposure from Able and Baker, Jim's tumor would have appeared either at a later date or not at all. Cause-in-fact is thereby established.

Theories of Liability of Toxic Waste Generators
Who Contaminate the Ambient Air

Society has an ongoing role of declaring and balancing interrelated rights and duties among parties. The "rights" protect one's person and property and confer certain privileges. The "duties" delineate one's responsibility when one's acts and omissions affect the rights of others.

Jim would claim a right, at least in his own home, to breathe air not contaminated with the carcinogenic waste of Able Chemical and Baker Chemical. Jim's remedy for an infringement of that right might be of an equitable nature, of a legal nature, or both. An injunction to prevent such contamination of the ambient air with known carcinogens would be characterized as an equitable remedy. Monetary damages for any proven harm from such contamination would be called a legal remedy. While society permits the toxic waste generator to discharge, at least to some extent, its carcinogenic waste into the environment, such a license does not insulate the TWG against liability for monetary damages to its toxic harm victims but merely protects it against certain equitable remedies such as injunctions. In resolving disputes involving harm from the interaction between "rights and duties," society can be said to play a role in the allocation of risks. In allocating risks, "strict liability" is applied in some situations. Thus the risk is placed on the party who causes the harm. The victim will still be required to prove certain facts, including legal causation, and the party causing the harm still has available certain defenses. Strict liability may be applicable to toxic harm caused by a TWG in some circumstances and not in others. The rules in identical situations often differ among the various states. This means that Jim may have an effective legal remedy in Texas but not in Louisiana. Differently stated, Able and Baker may be strictly liable to its toxic harm victims in one state but not in another. Of course, the balance of political power among the parties may affect the allocation of risks.

Several legal theories employ the strict liability concept. In our example involving contamination of Jackson's ambient air with carcinogens, strict liability theories would include trespass (an intentional invasion by a physical agent), some forms of nuisance, ultrahazardous activities, and what may be simply called a pollution tort for intentional invasions. In our example the word "intentional" would simply mean an awareness by Able and Baker that their activities necessarily involved the discharge of chemical waste into the ambient air. The trespass theory is an attractively simple remedy for contamination of the ambient air. In different states trespass has been both applied and rejected.[3] A principal inadequacy of "ultrahazardous activity" as a basis for strict liability lies in the uncertainty whether a given activity is to be deemed ultrahazardous. Such uncertainty could be reduced with a definition including all activities creating a foreseeable risk of toxic harm.

Where toxic harm is caused by the migration of a TWG's toxic waste through air or water, the law of nuisance is used most frequently to determine its responsibility, if any. Nuisance law is ordinarily invoked where one party uses his property (e.g., for the

---

3. *Martin v. Reynolds Metals Co.*, 221 Ore. 86, 342 P. 2d 790, 794 (1959), applying trespass theory; *Arvidson v. Reynolds Metals Co.*, 125 F. Suppl. 481 (S.D., Wash. 1954), rejecting trespass theory.

operation of a chemical plant) in a manner that disturbs another party in the use and enjoyment of his property. Some types of interference constitute a private nuisance as a matter of law (e.g., an interference prohibited by statute). Other types of interference may constitute a private nuisance only when deemed unreasonable (e.g., odors). Where reasonable people may differ on whether a given interference is unreasonable, the dispute will be resolved by the fact finder (e.g., jury). The consensus on reasonableness may differ in different areas.

If a TWG, in disposing of its toxic waste, interferes with the enjoyment and use of public property, a public nuisance may be found to exist. An individual can recover on the basis of a public nuisance only when his harm is different from that experienced by the general public. Liability based on nuisance may be affected by whether a release of toxic waste is intentional (e.g., for normal process, fugitive and storage emissions from a chemical plant) or unintentional (e.g., from an explosion). Court decisions are often inconsistent in describing the nature and scope of nuisance law and its application to given facts.

Referring again to our hypothetical case, we will assume that Jim's brain tumor was caused by Able and Baker's contaminating the ambient air with low-level doses of carcinogenic substances. Jim will claim that the invasion of his home with carcinogens unleashed by Able and Baker constituted an absolute nuisance with strict liability on their part for his resulting brain tumor. Moreover, Jim will claim that such carcinogenic contamination of Jackson's ambient air created a public nuisance resulting in special harm to him.

On the other hand, Able and Baker will point out that their operations have economic benefits for the city of Jackson and its residents; that their operations are in all respects lawful; that the public regulates, by issuing permits, the disposal of their toxic waste and that they have at all relevant times been in compliance with their permits; and that therefore they have acted as reasonable and prudent chemical companies in their release of carcinogenic substances into the ambient air of Jackson.

Negligence law is commonly used in balancing conflicting rights (or allocating risks) where one party, in the use of his property, causes harm to another. "Reasonableness" is the key concept in resolving such conflicts. Negligence is defined as the failure to exercise ordinary care—the care a prudent party would ordinarily exercise in the same or similar circumstances.

"Reasonable" persons may differ among themselves on whether certain conduct by a party is reasonable or unreasonable. Under negligence law a party is responsible only for the foreseeable consequences of his conduct. No liability attaches for consequences that are remote or inconceivable.

New technology and its effects often challenge the capacity of existing legal theories to resolve newly created conflicts. Usually a traditional theory is sufficiently adaptable, but sometimes a new theory will offer greater clarity and less confusion by directly addressing the conflict. An outstanding opinion in a Texas case formulated an express legal theory on harm from intentional air and water pollution.[4]

In factual disputes, the controlling facts must be determined by the judge or jury. A single set of facts may give rise to more than one legal basis of liability. Ordinarily a claimant can allege alternative facts and as many causes of action (legal theories proving remedies) as the alleged facts may confer.

What legal theories will Jim use against Able and Baker? Jim's first choice may be to ask that strict liability be applied for a pollution tort arising from harm caused by the intentional discharge of carcinogens into the ambient air. A second choice would be to contend that the disposal of carcinogenic waste is an ultrahazardous activity and that therefore strict liability attaches. A third choice would be for Jim to contend that Able and Baker committed a trespass by setting in motion carcinogenic waste, knowing that it would invade nearby homes, churches, schools, and other places where people had a right to be.[5] A fourth choice would be to argue that such contamination of the ambient air with carcinogenic substances created both a public and a private nuisance. A fifth basis of recovery against Able and Baker would be to claim that Jim's harm was caused by negligence on their part, particularly as to the nature and quantity of the carcinogenic waste showered on the town of Jackson.

Regardless of the legal theories used, Jim (through his attorney

---

4. *Atlas Chemical Industry, Inc., v. Anderson*, 514 S.W. 2d 309 (Tex. Civ. App. 1974) aff'd. 524 S.W. 2d 681 (Tex. 1975).

5. See note 3.

and experts) should identify and roughly quantify the carcinogenic waste of Able and Baker to which he was exposed and then
prove (more likely than not) that such exposure was a legal cause
of his brain tumor.

Finding a Lawyer for the Toxic Harm Victim

In most areas where toxic harm occurs, there will probably be one
or more lawyers who will have the experience, resources, and
motivation to handle any indicated litigation. Usually such a lawyer
will be available for a conference without cost or obligation to the
victim. If the damages are significant and there is a fair chance of
recovery, the lawyer will ordinarily be willing to take the case for
a contingent fee—he will receive as his fee an agreed percentage of
the recovery; if there is no recovery, then no fee is paid.

The lawyer chosen should have the experience and resources to
adequately handle personal injury and disease litigation and prefer-
ably should have experience in preparing and presenting evidence
to establish toxic exposure and evidence supporting a causal link
between that exposure and the plaintiff's harm. A lawyer with the
desired qualifications may be found through publicity, inquiries to
representatives of environmental organizations, or recommendations by knowledgeable courthouse workers. While not yet widely
employed, the most effective way of getting the victim and a qualified (and motivated) attorney together is advertising by the
attorney.

Some lawyers accept toxic harm claims and then refer the cases
to other lawyers who perform the work under an agreement whereby the fee is split. Since toxic claims are relatively new, complex,
and expensive, a lawyer will sometimes accept a case directly that
he would turn down as a referral. Therefore the victim may be
better served by contracting only with the lawyer who will perform all or a significant portion of the legal services.

How Did Things Get This Way?

The discussion of our hypothetical case illustrates the complexity
of litigating a toxic harm claim. Such complexity, together with the
enormous expense, explains why so few claims have been made.

We have allowed toxic waste generators (TWGs) to inflict, with
virtual impunity, toxic harm on millions of people as well as to do
inestimable environmental harm. Kept powerless by political inac-
tion, we for many years permitted our ambient air, surface water,

groundwater, and the good earth to be freely appropriated as random dump sites for toxic waste. When enough influential citizens sensed the ongoing harm and got a glimpse of the specter of a toxic avalanche with the potential for doing us all in, the public gained sufficient political strength for regulatory legislation. This legislation, as expected, was opposed by the TWGs, who apparently had come to view themselves as entitled to unleash their toxic waste into the environment without restraint.

As the evidence of toxic harm mounted and the potential consequences of the toxic avalanche became better perceived, more regulatory legislation was enacted to protect public health and the environment. While the public has greatly benefited from the major environmental laws, the TWGs have significantly reduced the laws' effectiveness with their vast legal and political resources. The TWGs, of course, do not want toxic harm to occur, but their concern for such harm remains subservient to their desire to generate and dispose of toxic waste with as little restraint and responsibility as possible.

We Expect Too Much of the Toxic Waste Generator

The toxic waste generator feels threatened by the discovery that its operations may contribute to disease. When vinyl chloride monomer became recognized as a carcinogen, the affected TWGs assumed a defensive adversary posture, minimizing the risk and opposing regulatory efforts by the federal government. The TWGs have done little to discover cancer morbidity or suggested reproductive harm among populations exposed to vinyl chloride monomer. Brain cancer has been suggested as a risk among petrochemical workers producing vinyl chloride, but this suggestion instantly prompted an adversary reaction by the affected TWGs, followed by their preparing rebuttal evidence from "proprietary" data.

The TWGs again and again have effectively resisted public regulations aimed at preventing toxic harm. They spent millions of dollars to fight reduced benzene exposure and recently have spent millions to weaken environmental regulations such as the Clean Air Act. Some TWGs have openly obstructed public investigations of cancer dangers to their own workers. In fact, the TWGs have even opposed efforts by their own workers to investigate disease dangers in the workplace. We, the public, have expected too much of the toxic waste generators.

It is naive to expect a serious effort by the TWGs to use part of their profits to discover disease dangers that would invite regulatory action and liability to their toxic harm victims. Through purposeful neglect, the TWG can promote ignorance and uncertainty about toxic harm. Such neglect, though not benign, is something the corporate entity can live with. The TWG is a private corporate entity. Its mission is profit, and it resists detracting factors. The public should realistically accept the TWG for what it is. Consistent with its corporate nature and mission, the TWG has made it abundantly clear that it wants an arrangement with society whereby the TWG has these rights: to engage in industrial activities creating risks of toxic harm; to unilaterally determine the acceptable levels of exposure to its toxic waste, thereby avoiding public regulation and interference; to avoid any penalty for breaching its common-law duty to discover disease dangers from its operations; to place the burden of toxic harm on the victims and the public; and to prevent others from discovering toxic harm by withholding information needed to compile exposure data, identify victims, and establish causal relations.

Once the public accepts the corporate nature of the TWG, we can proceed to fashion a plan offering some measure of protection against toxic harm and then, with much greater frequency, make the TWG responsible to its toxic harm victims.

A Proposal to Better Protect the Public

To better identify toxic harm and to allocate its costs, a special tax should be levied against the toxic waste generator to finance the public performance of its common-law duty. After all, creating risks of widespread toxic harm is not an absolute right, but rather a privilege that society can withhold or confer with reasonable conditions. One such condition should be compelling the TWG to disclose all information helpful in compiling exposure data on populations at risk and identifying toxic harm victims. Public health investigators should compile such exposure data and should conduct appropriate studies to ascertain any causal relation between such exposure and harm. If the public took over the TWG's common-law duty, data worthy of confidence would be created, and the TWG would be freed of a troublesome conflict of interest.

For the time being the TWG should be penalized, but fairly so, for having legally wronged its victims. One act of legal restitution would be for the courts to appoint masters, at the TWG's expense, to compile exposure data where there is reasonable basis for believing a plaintiff victim has sustained harm that may have been caused by toxic exposure created by the defendant TWG. Such exposure data, with appropriate modifications, could thereafter be utilized by other plaintiffs.

Because of its breach of duty, the TWG should be denied (estopped) use of the statute of limitations to defeat the legal rights of a victim or his beneficiaries. The breach of duty by the TWG has left plaintiffs with evidence problems in proving legal causation. Fairness would be served by applying judicial innovations as well as traditional legal tools such as presumptions to such evidence problems.

Conclusion

The burden of toxic harm will continue to increase for these reasons:

- The continuing generation of enormous quantities of toxic waste.
- The vast quantities of toxic waste currently in the environment, including innumerable dump sites where such waste is either doing its damage or is on standby, threatening harm.
- The many ultimate victims from past exposure where incipient, time-dependent disease is still evolving toward morbidity.
- The legacy of accumulating heritable mutations.

We are in dire need of a public strategy to reduce the burden of toxic harm and to do justice to the individual victims. Our society prides itself on concern for the individual, including the protection of his life, the integrity of his mind and body, and the defense of his property. This societal protection has been grossly inadequate to cope with the mounting toxic onslaught of the past thirty years.

We have failed to adequately identify the various forms of toxic harm, and we remain ignorant of its magnitude. We are not likely to secure better protection until we arm ourselves with the data necessary to reveal the nature and extent of this toxic harm. Of elementary importance (and the most neglected) is the necessary exposure data. Such data are needed to better identify the populations at risk, to improve the design of toxicity studies, and to enhance the design and evaluation of epidemiologic studies.

We, the public, have utterly failed our toxic harm victims. We have naively entrusted the TWGs to create and record vital exposure data and to properly study their employee populations at risk. Predictably, the TWGs have avoided programs to ascertain disease dangers. Identifying toxic dangers would only invite regulation liability. Instead the TWG, for its own economic protection, has used its resources to exonerate its accused chemicals.

I propose a new policy whereby dependable data would be created to effectively identify and prevent toxic harm. Such data would be created by public health personnel at TWG expense. The newly created data, together with a just, innovative judiciary would offer toxic harm victims legal relief with much greater frequency. The cost of toxic harm to the extent of such relief, plus the cost of creating the necessary data, would finally be properly allocated. Once the cost is fixed, the TWG, consistent with its purpose of profit, will more seriously undertake prevention measures to reduce its own financial burden.

10   Resource Guide

Earon S. Davis
Valerie A. Wilk

his resource guide lists further bibliographical and organizational resources so you can identify and pursue those that will be directly relevant to your particular interests and needs. The guide is divided into six subject areas, which are by no means mutually exclusive.

1. Background materials on toxic substances and the regulatory process
   A. General resources
   B. The right to know
   C. Industry
2. Health effects
   A. Computer searches
   B. Public health schools, medical schools, and universities and colleges
   C. Experts and testing laboratories
   D. Publications
   E. Libraries
3. Toxic substances and the law
4. Epidemiology and biostatistics
   A. Experts and organizations
   B. Publications
5. Risk assessment
6. Directories, guides, and catalogs

Reprinted by permission of the Farmworker Justice Fund, c/o Migrant Legal Action Program, 2001 S Street, NW, Washington, D.C. 20009

191

Some of these categories include information on organizations that might be able to provide advice on particular issues that concern you. The bulk of this guide, however, consists of annotated bibliographical references to publications dealing with some of the many issues related to toxic substances.

1. Background Materials on Toxic Substances and the Regulatory Process

A. General Resources

U.S. Environmental Protection Agency, Office of Pesticides and Toxic Substances. *Federal Activities in Toxic Substances.* Toxics Integration Information Series, EPA-560/13-80-015. Washington, D.C.: Environmental Protection Agency, 1980.

This 318 page book presents an overview of most government efforts and programs for controlling toxic substances. Agency and program descriptions include: Consumer Product Safety Commission, Council on Environmental Quality, Department of Agriculture, Department of Health and Human Services, Department of Labor, Department of Transportation, Environmental Protection Agency (ten listings), and National Toxicology Program. Topics discussed for each program include organization, statutory authorities, regulatory development, and toxics-related activities. Copies may be obtained from the Industry Assistance Office at the EPA, tel. (800) 424-9065 or (800) 554-1404.

Hazardous Substances in the Environment—Law and Policy. Special issue, *Ecology Law Quarterly* 7, no. 2 (1980):1-677.

A 677 page book, available for $5 from the School of Law, University of California, Berkeley, California 94720. Contains several excellent articles related to toxic substances:
Page, T. "A Generic View of Toxic Chemicals and Other Risks."
Freedman, D.M. "Reasonable Certainty of No Harm: Reviving the Safety Standard for Food Additives, Color Additives, and Animal Drugs."
Berger, J.L., and S.D. Riskin. "Economic and Technological Feasibility in Regulating Toxic Substances under the Occupational Safety and Health Act."
Slesin, L., and R. Sandler. "Categorization of Chemicals under the Toxic Substances Control Act."
Alston, P. "International Regulation of Toxic Chemicals."
Padway, L. "Federal Regulation of Ritalin in the Treatment of Hyperactive Children."
Doniger, D. "Federal Regulation of Vinyl Chloride: A Short Course in the Law and Policy of Toxic Substances Control."

Environmental Quality. Eleventh annual report. Washington, D.C.: Council on Environmental Quality, 1980: especially chap. 6, "Toxic Substances and Environmental Health."

An excellent introduction to the toxics problem. Topics covered include health effects (cancer, lung disease, reproduction), widespread exposures (e.g., lead, caffeine, diesels), waste disposal, Superfund, compensation of victims, trade secrets, and exports of hazardous substances. Other general treatments include those under the topics of chemical pollution (p. 56) and water quality (p. 85).

Environmental Quality. Tenth annual report. Washington, D.C.: Council on Environmental Quality, 1979.

Like its counterpart in the eleventh annual report, the chapter entitled "Toxic Substances and Environmental Health" (chap. 3) presents an excellent overview of the problems and the responses. This report, however, focuses on additional areas such as low-level radiation, dioxin, cotton dust, benzene, lead, saccharin, nitrites, residues, and toxics export policies under the EPA, Consumer Product Safety Commission, and Food and Drug Administration.

Commoner, Barry. *The Closing Circle: Nature, Man and Technology.* New York: Bantam Books, 1971.

A classic treatment of the concept of the human ecosystem and the fact that humans cannot survive unless they are aware of the consequences of their actions and responsible enough to choose life over short-term profits and conveniences.

Portney, Paul R., ed. *Current Issues in U.S. Environmental Policy.* Resources for the Future. Baltimore: Johns Hopkins University Press, 1978.

Portney, Paul R. "Toxic Substance Policy and the Protection of Human Health," chap. 4.

Peskin, Henry M. "Environmental Policy and the Distribution of Benefits and Costs," chap. 5.

Epstein, Samuel O., Lestor O. Brown, and Carl Pope. *Hazardous Waste in America.* San Francisco: Sierra Club Books, 1982.

An up-to-date 593 page overview and reference source for hazardous waste, including sections on case studies, the law, and problems and technologies. There is also an extensive appendix listing toxic waste generators, location of hazardous waste sites, a review of statutes, and other topics.

Boyle, Robert, and the Environmental Defense Fund. *Malignant Neglect.* New York: Knopf, 1970.

This book, primarily by Joseph L. Highland, Marcia E. Fine, and Robert H. Boyle, is an authoritative report on known or suspected cancer-causing agents in our environment and how, by controlling them, we can control the spread of cancer itself.

Epstein, Samuel S. *The Politics of Cancer.* San Francisco: Sierra Club Books, 1978.

This powerful book presents scientific evidence of the cancer epidemic and describes the ways government responses to the problem have been limited and ineffective.

Public Opinion on Environmental Issues: Results of a National Public Opinion Survey. Washington, D.C.: U.S. Government Printing Office, 1980.

This report presents the results of the 1980 survey conducted by Resources for the Future for the EPA, the U.S. Department of Agriculture, the Department of Energy, and the Council on Environmental Quality. The survey revealed a strong public commitment to paying the price necessary to protect health and the environment. The public concern over the toxic chemical waste problem surpassed the level of concern for any other environmental problem within the past decade.

Gusman, S., K. von Moltke, F. Irwin, and C. Whitehead. *Public Policy for Chemicals: National and International Issues.* Washington, D.C.: Conservation Foundation, 1980.

An international effort to address the problems of toxic chemicals. Topics include assessing hazards, notification requirements, risk assessment and control, international trade, transfer of information, and policy options.

Toxic Chemicals and Public Protection. A report to the president by the Toxic Substances Strategy Committee, 1980.

This committee report discusses the current federal activities involving research on and regulation of toxic chemicals. The multiagency task force (chaired by Gus Speth) recommended strengthening these federal efforts to protect the public from exposure to toxic chemicals. Topics discussed are chemical information systems, confidentiality, research, emergency response, regulatory programs, cancer policy, and international issues.

"Toxics in the New Jersey Environment: Microcosm of United States Ills." *Civil Engineering* (American Society of Civil Engineers), September 1979, pp. 74–78.

Discusses toxics in the context of New Jersey but is applicable to any area. Topics discussed include toxics in the groundwater, surface water, and air as well as environmental concerns and the hazardous waste problem.

Nader, Ralph, Ronald Brownstein, and John Richard, eds. *Who's Poisoning America: Corporate Polluters and Their Victims in the Chemical Age.* San Francisco: Sierra Club Books, 1981.

This 369 page book is a compilation of seven specific toxic chemical incidents across the country: PBB in Michigan, kepone in Virginia, nuclear wastes in West Valley, New York, PCBs in the Hudson River, mine tailings in Lake Superior, 2,4,5-T in northern California, and the hazardous wastes of Love Canal.

A Toxics Primer. Publication 545. Washington, D.C.: League of Women Voters Education Fund, 1979.

This pamphlet presents an excellent overview of the toxics problem.

Toxic Substances: A Brief Overview of the Issues Involved. Washington, D.C.: Environmental Protection Agency, 1980.

Prepared by the New Jersey Public Interest Research Group and New Jersey League of Women Voters. Issues discussed include biology, chemistry, physiology, analysis (risk), and law. There is an extensive bibliography.

The Toxic Substances Dilemma. Washington, D.C.: National Wildlife Federation, 1980.

This excellent document presents a background on toxic chemicals and their health effects. Focusing on toxic substances discharged into the environment, it discusses what the federal government is doing and how citizens can take action.

"Toxic Substances: EPA and OSHA Are Reluctant Regulators." *Science* 203 (5 January 1979): 28.

Discusses some of the institutional problems in regulating toxic substances.

"Those Toxic Chemical Wastes." *Time,* 22 September 1980.

This cover story discusses the toxic waste problem and tells what is being done about it.

Kunofsky, J. *Training Materials on Toxic Substances: Tools for Effective Action.* San Francisco: Sierra Club Books, 1981.

These materials, funded by the EPA and printed by the Sierra Club, contain a great deal of information and advice on how to form and maintain a grassroots environmental organization.

"Waste Alert." Special issue of *Environmental Protection Agency Journal,* vol. 5, no. 2 (February 1979).

Explores, through numerous separate articles, the problems and responses resulting from toxic chemical wastes. "Waste Alert" was a program by which the EPA worked toward informing the public of the hazards involving solid and toxic wastes.

Agran, Larry. *The Cancer Connection.* New York: St. Martin's Press, 1977.

Presents the personal stories of several people with environmentally induced cancers and discusses the societal implications of the ways cancer can be— but is not being—prevented.

"Clean Air Special." Special issue of *Amicus Journal* 2, no. 3 (Winter 1981).

Published by the Natural Resources Defense Council. See the following items:

Ronald Brownstein. "Ronald Reagan's Washington" (discussion of toxic chemicals), p. 7

David Doniger. "The Growing Threat from Toxic Chemical Air Pollutants," pp. 26–27.

Anthony D. Cortese. "The Health Basis for Clean Air," pp. 28–32.

David Doniger. "Hold Your Breath: The Diesels Are Coming," pp. 33–34.

Ashford, Nicholas. *Crisis in the Workplace.* Cambridge: Ford Foundation, MIT Press, 1976.

Discussion of the following areas is included: nature and dimensions of the problem, the Occupational Safety and Health Act, states, economics, workers' compensation, and agricultural workers.

Damages and Threats Caused by Hazardous Material Sites. EPA 430/9-80-004, WH-548. Washington, D.C.: U.S. Environmental Protection Agency, Oil and Special Materials Control Division, 1980.

A partial compilation of data readily available to the EPA during February and March of 1980. Presents information on damage and threats of damage by more than 350 hazardous waste sites in the United States. Damage includes groundwater contamination, drinking water well closures, fish kills, property damage from fires and explosions, and kidney disorders, cancer, and death. Available from Environmental Action Foundation, Waste and Toxic Substances Project, 724 Dupont Circle Building, Washington, D.C. 20036, tel. (202) 296-7570.

Danger in the Field: The Myth of Pesticide Safety. Immokalee: Florida Rural Legal Services, 1980.

This 53 page report resulted from a study of the extent of farmworker exposure to pesticides in southern Florida. It also evaluates the efficiency of the EPA's Pesticide Incident Monitoring System (PIMS). Findings include that PIMS is inadequate for determining the actual numbers of pesticide poisonings, that the pesticide hazard is widespread, and that pesticide laws are not well enforced.

Ground Water Protection: A Water Quality Management Report. SW-886. Washington, D.C.: Environmental Protection Agency, Water Planning Division, 1980.

Explores the issues surrounding threats to groundwater in the United States.

It includes several articles discussing groundwater pollution and availability, the role of hazardous wastes and other sources of groundwater pollution, and what is being done about solving the problems.

Hazardous Materials Transportation Accident Statistics and Emergency Response Problems. Waste and Toxic Substances Project, Information Packet T-1. Washington, D.C.: Environmental Action Foundation, 1980.

Hazardous Waste Facility Siting: A Critical Problem. SW-865. Washington, D.C.: Environmental Protection Agency, 1980.

Discusses the critical shortage of hazardous waste disposal sites and the problems involved in site selection and public opposition.

Hunt the Dump. Environmental Action and the Sierra Club, n.p., n.d.

This 8 page publication, reprinted by the National Wildlife Federation, presents a campaign to locate and expose the nation's unsafe hazardous waste sites. It discusses the toxic dump problem and then presents citizen action tools for helping to clean up (and prevent) problems.

Indoor Air Pollution: An Emerging Health Problem. U.S. Comptroller General Report to the Congress of the United States. Washington, D.C.: U.S. Government Accounting Office, 1980.

Finds that there is not adequate government response to the growing evidence that indoor air pollution presents a significant public health problem. Recommends that one agency, the EPA, be given indoor air authority under Clean Air Act amendments.

Brown, Michael. *Laying Waste: The Poisoning of America by Toxic Chemicals.* New York: Pantheon Books, 1980.

Michael Brown is the journalist who exposed the frightening Love Canal story. In this book he presents the story behind the situation at and around Love Canal as well as numerous other toxic time bombs throughout the United States.

Weir, David, and Mark Shapiro. *Circle of Poison.* San Francisco: Institute for Food and Development Policy, 1981.

Documents the international sales of the most deadly pesticides and tells how they return to the United States via imported foods. Pesticides banned in the United States can still be manufactured here and exported to Third World nations, where their use is virtually unregulated.

Gibbs, Lois. *Love Canal: My Story.* Albany: State University of New York Press, 1982.

Tells the story of how "average" citizens were able to force the government to recognize and take action regarding serious health problems caused by a hazardous waste dump.

Van der Bosch, Robert. *The Pesticide Conspiracy.* New York: Anchor Books, 1980.

Chronicles the ways the chemical industry has influenced both the scientific research process and government regulation of pesticides.

Carson, Rachel. *Silent Spring.* Greenwich, Conn.: Crest Books, 1962.

This is the book that ignited the environmental movement of the 1960s. It revealed the ubiquity of deadly chemicals in the human environment and warned that disaster would follow if current trends were not reversed. Needless to say, the warning was not heeded.

Regenstein, Lewis. *America the Poisoned.* Washington, D.C.: Acropolis Books, 1982.

This 414 page book presents an important overview of the abuse of pesticides and other deadly chemicals in our society. Chapters discuss herbicide use, pesticides, toxic wastes, water and air pollution, export of toxics, and health hazards. Specific chapters explore Tris, PCBs, lindane, DBCP, endrin, toxaphene, DDT, aldrin and dieldrin, and chlordane and heptachlor.

Health Hazards for Office Workers. Cleveland: Working Women Education Fund, 1981.

This excellent 57 page booklet describes the basic health hazards that office workers are subject to. These range from job stress and long working hours to noise, improper lighting, inadequate ventilation, air quality problems, and toxic chemical exposures as well as other safety and fire hazards. It is available for $4 from Working Women Education Fund, 1224 Huron Road, Cleveland, Ohio 44115.

NCAP News 1, no. 4 (Winter/Spring 1980).

This quarterly publication of the Northwest Coalition for Alternatives to Pesticides presents a great deal of information on topics such as scientific studies, citizen action techniques, national pesticide news, local events, and how to avoid use of pesticides. NCAP also has available other information packets, literature, and technical reports. The address is NCAP News, Box 375, Eugene, Oregon 97440.

Pesticide Use and Misuse: Farmworkers and Small Farmers Speak on the Problem. Rural American Report. Washington, D.C.: Rural America, 8 September 1980.

Presents the views of farmworkers on the nature and extent of pesticide problems they are facing.

Sierra (Sierra Club Bulletin), 66, no. 2 (March/April 1981).

See the following items:
Stoler, Peter. "Is Clean Water a Thing of the Past?" pp. 14–18.

Miller, Mark, and Judith Miller. "Detecting Cancer," pp. 19-22.

Roeder, Edward. "Catalyzing Favorable Reactions: A Look at Chemical Industry's PAC's," pp. 23-26.

McCloskey, Michael. "Environmental Protection Is Good Business," pp. 31-33.

Moss, Larry E. "Beyond Conflict: The Art of Environmental Mediation," pp. 40-45.

"The Sierra Club and Toxic Substances," staff report, pp. 66-70.

Siting of Hazardous Waste Management Facilities and Public Opposition. SW-809. Washington, D.C.: Environmental Protection Agency, 1979.

Presents several case studies of problems faced in siting hazardous waste management facilities.

Hazardous Waste: A Community Action Guide. Washington, D.C.: Concern, Inc., 1981.

This good introduction to community action on hazardous waste issues (22 pages) is available for $3 from Concern, Inc., 1794 Columbia Rd., NW, Washington, D.C. 20009, tel. (202) 328-8160

Siting of Hazardous Waste Management Facilities and Public Opposition. SW-Women Voters of the U.S., n.d.

This pamphlet may be ordered for 35 cents from League of Women Voters of the U.S., 1730 M Street, NW, Washington, D.C. 20036.

Keystone Process Siting Group. *Siting Waste Management Facilities in the Galveston Bay Area: A New Approach.* Keystone, Colo.: Keystone Center, 1982.

A 50 page report from the Keystone Workshops on siting nonradioactive hazardous waste management facilities. Available from the Keystone Center, box 38, Keystone, Colorado 80435.

Courrier, Kathleen, ed. *Life after '80: Environmental Choices We Can Live With.* Andover, Mass.: Center for Renewable Resources, Brick House Publishing Company, 1980.

This 280 page book presents a series of practical essays on environmental and energy issues facing us in the present and the near future.

Kamlet, Kenneth S. *Toxic Substances Programs in U.S. States and Territories: How Well Do They Work?* Scientific and Technical Series 4. Washington, D.C.: National Wildlife Federation, 1979.

This 21 page pamphlet surveys the laws in each state regarding toxic chemicals. While the results present a good picture of the state efforts before the federal programs under the Resources Conservation and Recovery Act and the Toxic Substances Control Act, it is important to secure more current data before using these figures.

Requirements of Laws and Regulations Enforced by the U.S. Food and Drug Administration. HEW Publication 79-1042. Rockville, Md.: U.S. Department of Health, Education and Welfare, Public Health Service, FDA, 1979.

B. The Right to Know

Friedland, John. "The Challenge of Informing Workers of Job-Related Health Hazards." In *Toxic Substances and Hazardous Wastes.* ALI-ABA Course of Study Materials. Washington, D.C.: Environmental Law Institute, 1980.

Gusman, Sam, and Frances Irwin. *Chemical Hazard Warnings: Labeling for Effective Communication.* Washington, D.C.: Conservation Foundation, 1979.

This 28 page issue report discusses the various aspects of developing effective labels for chemicals so that intelligent decisions can be made regarding their use. The report discusses the purposes of labels, emphasizing those in the workplace. An appendix presents various labeling laws such as the Toxic Substances Control Act, Occupational Safety and Health Act, Consumer Product Safety Act, Food, Drug, and Cosmetic Act, and Federal Insecticide, Fungicide, and Rodenticide Act, as well as voluntary industrial practices. For Conservation Foundation publications the address is 1717 Massachusetts Avenue, NW, Washington, D.C. 20036.

The Right to Know: Practical Problems and Policy Issues Arising from Exposures to Hazardous Chemicals and Physical Agents in the Workplace. Washington, D.C.: National Institute for Occupational Safety and Health, Center for Disease Control, Public Health Service, U.S. Department of Health, Education, and Welfare, 1977.

Hunt, V. "The Emergence of the Worker's Right to Know Health Risks." In *Strategies for Public Health,* ed. L. K. Y. Ng and D. L. Davis, chap. 11. New York: Van Nostrand Reinhold, 1981.

Weiner, Peter H. "The Right to Know: Toxic Substances and the Workplace." In *Toxic Substances and Hazardous Wastes.* ALI-ABA Course of Study Materials. Washington, D.C.: Environmental Law Institute, 1980.

Right to Know. Waste and Toxic Substances Project, Information Packet 1-1, Legislation. Washington, D.C.: Environmental Action Foundation, 1980.

C. Industry

Moskowitz, M., M. Katz, and R. Levering. *Everybody's Business: An Almanac. The Irreverent Guide to Corporate America.* San Francisco: Harper and Row, 1980.

This 916 page book is packed with interesting and useful information about corporations in America and what they have been up to. $9.95.

A Challenge to Fear (the Facts about Cancer in the U.S.A.). Midland, Mich.: Dow Chemical Company, 1978.

Available free from Dow Chemical U.S.A., Health and Environmental Research, Midland, Michigan 48640.

Chemical Product Safety: What We're Doing about It. Washington, D.C.: Chemical Manufacturers Association, n.d.

Available free from Chemical Manufacturers Association, 1825 Connecticut Avenue NW, Washington, D.C. 20009.

A Closer Look at the Pesticide Question for Those Who Want the Facts. Midland, Mich.: Dow Chemical Company, 1981.

Available free from Dow Chemical U.S.A., Health and Environmental Research, Midland, Michigan 48640.

Exxon USA 19, no. 3 (third quarter 1980), Houston, Texas.

Exxon USA 19, no. 4 (fourth quarter 1980), Houston, Texas.

Protecting the Environment: What We're Doing about It. Washington, D.C.: Chemical Manufacturers Association, n.d.

Available free from Chemical Manufacturers Association, 1825 Connecticut Avenue, NW, Washington, D.C. 20009.

A Review of Chemical Industry Economics and Statistics. Waste and Toxic Substances Project Information Packet B-1. Washington, D.C.: Environmental Action Foundation, 1980.

Lewert, Henry. *Silent Autumn.* Midland, Mich.: Dow Chemical Company, 1977.

Available free from Dow Chemical U.S.A., Midland, Michigan 48640.

Who Protects Our Health and Environment? Midland, Mich.: Toxicology Research Laboratory, Dow Chemical Company, 1980.

Available free from Dow Chemical U.S.A., Health and Environmental Research, Midland, Michigan 48640.

2. Health Effects

A. *Computer Searches*

When a bibliography of health-related information is needed, a time-saving device is the MEDLARS system. The National Library of Medicine (NLM) in Bethesda, Maryland, operates this computerized system (Medical Literature Analysis and Retrieval System), which contains some 4,500,000 references to journal articles and books on the health sciences published since 1965. MEDLARS is available at more than 1,300 universities, medical schools, hospitals, government agencies, and commercial organizations throughout the country, which connect with the NLM computers by telephone.

The "on-line" searches allow the user to "talk" to the computer to obtain the most relevant information. At some centers a librarian will do the search; at others the user will receive some preliminary instruction and run the search himself or herself. The NLM catalog of subject headings and key words that might appear in titles of abstracts is used to structure the search strategy. Once connection with the NLM computer has been made, the dialogue can be tailored to explore other areas if the original strategy is not proving fruitful. An on-line search produces a printout listing titles of articles and books, with the names of the authors and, for articles, the journal titles. If the requester wishes, an abstract of each article can also be printed. If a search yields a long bilbiography, the printout can be done off line at NLM and mailed out the next day to save time and money.

Some of the most useful on-line data bases for health and toxicology information are the following.

MEDLINE

MEDLINE contains references to biomedical journal articles. This data base will yield journal articles on results of epidemiologic and animal studies as well as information on human health effects. MEDLINE contains references for the current year and two preceding years, but off-line searches of back files (to 1966) can also be conducted.

TOXLINE

TOXLINE (Toxicology Information On Line) provides information on published human and animal toxicity studies, effects of environmental chemicals and pollutants, and adverse drug reactions. The on-line collection indexes references from the last five years. TOXBACK files contain information to 1965.

RTECS

The RTECS (Registry of Toxic Effects of Chemical Substances) data base contains acute toxicity data for approximately 41,000 substances. For some of the compounds information is included on threshold limit values, recommended standards in air, and aquatic toxicity.

TDB

TDB (Toxicology Data Bank) contains chemical, pharmacological, and toxicological information and data on approximately two thousand substances.

CANCERLIT

The CANCERLIT (Cancer Literature) data base deals exclusively with aspects of cancer.

CANCERPROJ

CANCERPROJ (Cancer Research Projects) contains descriptions of twenty thousand ongoing cancer research projects from the current year and two preceding years. These projects are being conducted throughout the world.

CHEMLINE

The CHEMLINE (Chemical Dictionary On-Line) data base is a file of names for chemical substances. It contains such information as the Chemical Abstracts Services registry numbers, molecular formulas, preferred chemical nomenclature, and generic and common names of substances.

B. *Public Health Schools, Medical Schools, and Universities and Colleges*

Besides written materials, another valuable source of information on a wide range of health and scientific issues is the academic community. Both faculty and professional staff researchers at universities, medical school, schools of public health, and colleges can be consulted.

Public Health Schools

Public health schools generally contain divisions of epidemiology, biostatistics or biometry, and environmental health. There are currently twenty-two schools of public health in the United States:

University of Alabama at Birmingham
Boston University, Boston
University of California, Berkeley
University of California, Los Angeles
Columbia University, New York
Harvard University, Boston
University of Hawaii, Honolulu
University of Illinois, Chicago
Johns Hopkins University, Baltimore
Loma Linda University, Loma Linda, California
University of Massachusetts, Amherst
University of Michigan, Ann Arbor
University of Minnesota, Minneapolis
University of North Carolina, Chapel Hill
University of Oklahoma, Oklahoma City
University of Pittsburgh, Pittsburgh
University of Puerto Rico, San Juan
University of South Carolina, Columbia
University of Texas, Houston
Tulane University, New Orleans
University of Washington, Seattle
Yale University, New Haven

Medical Schools

Universities with medical schools but not public health schools are also engaged in public health and epidemiologic research. In these schools the college of medicine generally contains a department of preventive medicine or of family or community medicine. Within such departments there are divisions of epidemiology, biostatistics, environmental health, health services administration, and other similar areas.

Universities and Colleges

Even if a local university or college does not have a medical school, faculty in science and mathematics departments may often be of help. Questions concerning biology, chemistry and toxicology, and statistics, for example, may be resolved by talking to professors in those departments. If local resource people cannot answer a specific question, they may know of colleagues who can or know where pertinent research is being conducted.

C. Experts and Testing Laboratories

Local resource people at medical schools, schools of public health, universities, and colleges (see above)

State health department

State environmental department

Private laboratories and research institutes in your area

Topical Directory. A-1907, OPA 120/9. Washington, D.C.: U.S. Environmental Protection Agency, Office of Public Awareness, 1980.

This directory of EPA personnel is divided into substantive areas of research or program activities. For each area, a principal contact is given, with a phone number.

Experts List. Washington, D.C.: Environmental Action Foundation, Waste and Toxic Substances Project, 1981.

The EAF maintains information on experts available to advise and assist citizens in areas related to toxic substances. The list is available from Environmental Action Foundation, 724 Dupont Circle Building, Washington, D.C. 20036, tel. (202) 296-7570.

Contact: Toxics—A Guide to Specialists on Toxic Substances. New York: World Environment Center.

Lists the names, telephone numbers, and professional profiles of almost a thousand specialists involved in the manufacture, handling, and disposal of toxic substances. Available for $37.50 for nonprofit organizations ($49.50 for government and industry) from World Environment Center, 300 East 42d Street, New York, New York 10017, tel. (212) 697-3232.

Publications List. The Environmental Defense Fund, 1525 Eighteenth Street, NW, Washington, D.C. 20036, tel. (202) 883-1484.

This organization puts out a publication list that includes reports, comments, petitions, pleadings, and so forth, prepared by their Toxic Chemicals Program.

Directory of Federal Coordinating Groups for Toxic Substances. 2d ed. Toxics Integration Information Series, EPA-560/13-80-008. Washington, D.C.: Environmental Protection Agency, 1980.

Includes names, addresses, and telephone numbers of federal, state, non-profit, and private-sector members of federal toxic chemical coordinating groups. International coordinating groups are not listed.

Registry. Arlington, Va.: Citizens Clearinghouse for Hazardous Wastes.

Founded by Lois Gibbs of Love Canal, Citizens Clearinghouse for Hazardous Wastes attempts to assist citizens across the country with hazardous waste problems. P.O. box 926, Arlington, Virginia 22216, tel. (703) 276-7070.

International Agency for Research on Cancer (IARC), Lyons, France.

Publishes a series of monographs and other scientific publications on a wide variety of cancer-related topics.

D. Publications

Rom, William N., ed. *Environmental and Occupational Medicine.* Boston: Little, Brown, 1983.

This new medical text is the most authoritative, complete, and well referenced work in its field. In addition to medical matters, chapters address legal and policy matters related to both environmental and occupational hazards. If you are looking for one authoritative book on "health effects," this is it.

Waldbott, George L. *Health Effects of Environmental Pollutants.* 2d ed. St. Louis: C. B. Mosby Company, 1978.

This 350 page paperback is perhaps the best work available on the health effects of pollutants, largely because it is readable and covers a wide range of pollutants.

Key, Marcus, Austin F. Henschel, Jack Butler, Robert N. Ligo, Irving Tabershaw, and Lorice Ede, eds. *Occupational Diseases: A Guide to Their Recognition.* Rev. ed. Washington, D.C.: U.S. Department of Health, Education, and Welfare, 1977.

This is the National Institute for Occupational Safety and Health standard text on occupational diseases. It is helpful in discussing the basic types of occupational diseases and then presenting the diseases related to various specific chemicals. Most helpful is a chart that states the occupational hazards for each category of industrial worker.

A Pocket Guide to Chemical Hazards. G8-210. Washington, D.C.: National Institute for Occupational Safety and Health, 1978.

This extremely useful booklet contains descriptions of the symptoms produced by hundreds of specific toxic chemicals studied by NIOSH and OSHA.

"A Brief Review of Selected Environmental Contamination Incidents with a Potential for Health Effects." Congressional Research Service of the Library of Congress, August 1980. In *Committee Print of the Senate Committee on Environment and Public Works,* serial no. 96–15. Washington, D.C.: U.S. Government Printing Office, 1980.

Health Hazards of the Human Environment. Geneva: World Health Organization, 1972.

A comprehensive overview of the various health hazards of the human environment, including toxic chemicals in the air, water, and food. It is helpful in developing an awareness of the interrelatedness of environmental problems and expanding the view of the human environment to include biological disease agents, overcrowding, crime, and other aspects of the human ecosystem.

Sartwell, Philip E. *Preventive Medicine and Public Health.* 10th ed. New York: Appleton-Century-Crofts, 1973.

Comprehensive (1,189 page) text covering a number of public health issues, including epidemiology (infectious and chronic diseases), environmental and occupational health, milk and food sanitation, water supplies, and waste disposal.

Zenz, Carl, ed. *Occupational Medicine: Principles and Practical Applications.* Chicago: Year Book Medical Publishers, 1975.

Comprehensive medical text on occupational health and diseases.

Randolph, Theron G. *Human Ecology and Susceptibility to the Chemical Environment.* Springfield, Ill.: Charles C. Thomas, 1962.

This pioneering work describes the ways individuals may become susceptible to chemicals in their environment, setting off a wide range of disease symptoms. Dr. Randolph is still treating patients with these same problems. He feels that the increasing exposures to all types of chemicals in our society is resulting in many more cases of hypersusceptibility, or chemical sensitivities, which can cause a variety of serious illnesses.

Ng, Lorenz K. Y., and Devra Lee Davis, eds. *Strategies for Public Health: Promoting Health and Preventing Disease.* New York: Van Nostrand Reinhold, 1981.

Kurzel, R. B., and C. L. Cetrulo. "The Effects of Environmental Pollutants on Human Reproduction, Including Birth Defects." *Environmental Science and Technology* 15, no. 6 (June 1981): 626–39.

This review article discusses the field of teratology as related to air pollutants, food additives, polyhalogenated biphenols, pesticides, metals and inorganic compounds, and other concerns. Published by the American Chemical Society.

Chemical Hazards to Human Reproduction. Washington, D.C.: Council on Environmental Quality, 1980.

Hayes, Wayland, Jr. *Toxicology of Pesticides.* Baltimore: Williams and Wilkins, 1975.

This 580 page text considers such subjects as dosage and other factors influencing toxicity, metabolism, nature of injuries and tests for them, pesticide studies in humans, recognized and possible exposure to pesticides, recognized and possible effects of pesticides in humans, domestic animals, and wildlife, diagnosis and treatment of poisoning, and prevention of injury by pesticides.

1981 Cancer Facts and Figures. New York: American Cancer Society, 1980.

A 31 page booklet available from American Cancer Society, 777 Third Avenue, New York, New York 10017.

Does Everything Cause Cancer? A Food Safety Primer. Washington, D.C.: Center for Science in the Public Interest, 1979.

This 12 page booklet answers questions people ask most about saccharin, nitrites, animal studies, and present food safety laws. It is available for $1 from Center of Science in the Public Interest, 1755 S Street, NW, Washington, D.C. 20009.

Environmental Cancer: Causes, Victims, Solutions. 2d ed. Summary of proceedings of a conference held 21 and 22 March 1977 by Urban Environment Conference. Washington, D.C., 1980.

Farm Chemicals Handbook, 1981. Willoughby, Ohio: Meister Publishing Company, 1981.

Published annually by *Farm Chemicals* magazine. It is primarily a directory and reference for the fertilizer and pesticide industries. Contains a pesticide dictionary, buyer's guide, plant food dictionary, and fertilizer trade names. The publisher is at 37841 Euclid Avenue, Willoughby, Ohio 44094.

Effects of Pesticides on the Immune Response. EPA-600. Washington, D.C.: U.S. Environmental Protection Agency, Health Effects Research Laboratory, 1979.

Recognition and Management of Pesticide Poisonings. 2d ed. Washington, D.C.: U.S. Environmental Protection Agency Office of Pesticide Programs, 1977.

Davies, John E. *Pesticide Protection: A Training Manual for Health Personnel.* Washington, D.C.: U.S. Department of Health, Education, and Welfare and U.S. Environmental Protection Agency Pesticide Office, 1977.

Pesticides: Fact Sheet. Washington, D.C.: Environmental Action Foundation (revised periodically).

Available from Environmental Action Foundation, Waste and Toxic Substances Project, 724 Dupont Circle Building, Washington, D.C. 20036, tel. (202) 296-7570.
The EAF maintains a mailing list for those interested in toxic chemicals, including pesticides. They also have several other publications of interest.

National Study of Hospitalized Pesticide Poisonings, 1974-76. Washington, D.C.: U.S. Environmental Protection Agency, 1980.

NAFP Pesticide Desk Reference. 2d draft. Washington, D.C.: National Association of Farmworker Organizations, 1980.

The Human Ecologist, Herbicide and Pesticide Impact Issue. Chicago: Human Ecology Action League, 1980.
See the following articles in this 12 page booklet:
Morgan, Joseph T. "Health Effects of Herbicides."
Randolph, Theron G. "Pesticides and Individual Susceptibility."
Larson, June. "Pesticide Update."

Cancer and the Worker. New York: New York Academy of Sciences, 1977.

Occupational Lung Diseases: An Introduction. New York: American Lung Association, 1979.
This excellent 80 page introduction to lung diseases is available from your local Lung Association affiliate.

Occupational Injuries and Illnesses in 1978: Summary. Report 586. Washington, D.C.: U.S. Department of Labor, Bureau of Labor Statistics, 1980.

Chemicals Identified in Human Biological Media, a Data Base: Second Annual Report. Bethesda, Md.: Interagency Collaborative Group on Environmental Carcinogenesis, National Cancer Institute, National Institutes of Health, 1980.
Available through the National Technical Information Service. Project Officer, Cindy Stroup, Exposure and Evaluation Division of EPA's Office of Pesticides and Toxic Substances, Washington, D.C. 20460, tel. (202) 755-8294. Volume 2, parts 1 and 2 present the entire data base of the project organized in several different manners, such as by chemical name, author, and chemical identification number.

Center for Science in the Public Interest. *The Household Pollutants Guide.* Garden City, N.Y.: Anchor Books/Doubleday, 1978.

Keough, Carol. *Water Fit to Drink.* Emmaus, Pa.: Rodale Press, 1980.
This paperback book discusses the problem of drinking-water contamination, explaining the alternative ways to purify drinking water and their relative effectiveness.

Health Aspects Related to Indoor Air Quality: Report on a World Health Organization Working Group, Copenhagen: Regional Office for Europe, 1979.

Damages and Threats Caused by Hazardous Material Sites. EPA 430/9-80-044, WH-548. Washington, D.C.: U.S. Environmental Protection Agency, Oil and Special Materials Control Division, 1980.

A partial compilation of data readily available to the EPA during February and March of 1980. Presents information on damage and threats of damage posed by more than 350 hazardous waste sites in the United States. Damage discussed includes groundwater contamination, drinking water well closures, fish kills, property damage from fires and explosions, and kidney disorders, cancer, and death. Available from Environmental Action Foundation, Waste and Toxic Substances Project, 724 Dupont Circle Building, Washington, D.C. 20036, tel (202) 296-7570.

Smith, A. *Managing Hazardous Substances Accidents.* New York: McGraw-Hill Book Company, 1981.

A manual written for the "first responder" to the hazardous substances accident (firefighter, civil defense officer, etc.). Available for $19.95 from McGraw-Hill Book Company, 1221 Avenue of the Americas, New York, New York 10020, tel (212) 997-3493.

U.S. Surgeon General. *Health Effects of Toxic Pollution: A Report from the Surgeon General and a Brief Review of Selected Environmental Contamination Incidents with a Potential for Health Effects.* Congressional Research Service of the Library of Congress, Report to the U.S. Senate Committee on Environment and Public Works. Serial no. 96-15. Washington, D.C.: U.S. Government Printing Office, 1980.

This report includes two documents: a 125 page report prepared by the Subcommittee on the Potential Health Effects of Toxic Chemical Dumps of the Department of Health and Human Services Committee to Coordinate Environmental and Related Programs and a 153 page report by the Congressional Research Service. The latter reviews the health implications of twenty-six specific substances and briefly describes six hazardous waste site incidents.

Randolph, Theron G., and Ralph W. Moss. *An Alternative Approach to Allergies.* New York: Harper and Row, 1980.

This 311 page book provides the theory behind the detection and treatment of environmental illness through clinical ecology. Dr. Randolph believes that chemical contaminants are causing a wide range of physical and emotional disorders in many individuals.

Calabrese, Edward J. *Pollutants and High-Risk Groups: The Biological Basis of Increased Human Susceptibility to Environmental and Occupational Pollutants.* New York: Wiley-Interscience, 1978.

This 266 page book discusses both proven and potential explanations for the tremendous variability in humans' susceptibility to adverse health effects from chemical pollutants. Susceptibility factors include human developmental factors (e.g., age, sex), genetic disorders, nutritional deficiencies, other disease conditions, and life-style (e.g., smoking, drug use).

Small, Bruce, *The Susceptibility Report*. Longueuil, Quebec: DECO-PLAN, 1982.

Discusses hazards caused by chemicals released in your home from building materials. The author presents the case against urea formaldehyde foam insulation, describing the serious potential health effects of formaldehyde in susceptible persons. Also discussed are remedial measures.

Whiteside, Thomas. *The Pendulum and the Toxic Cloud: The Course of Dioxin Contamination*. New Haven: Yale University Press, 1979.

Medical Journals

The following medical journals regularly report the results of studies of the health effects of occupational exposures or of exposure to toxic substances among the general public. These journals are found in medical school and hospital libraries.

American Journal of Epidemiology
Journal of Occupational Medicine
Archives of Environmental Health
American Public Health Association Journal
Clinical Toxicology
Regulatory Toxicology and Pharmacology

A new journal (vol. 1, 1981) that covers scientific and legal concepts concerning human health and the environment.

E. Libraries

The U.S. Environmental Protection Agency in Washington, D.C., has a library with an extensive collection of journals, books, and government publications on toxic substances and environmental issues. In addition, each of the ten EPA regional offices also has a library. These offices are in Boston, New York, Philadelphia, Atlanta, Chicago, Dallas, Kansas City, Missouri, Denver, San Francisco, and Seattle (see table 8.1 for addresses).

3. Toxic Substances and the Law

Published resources on toxic chemical laws are listed below. There are also several important organizational resources that should be considered, regarding both periodical information services and more individualized services. For example, the Association of Trial Lawyers of America (ATLA) offers its members a research service and brief bank through its Products Liability/ Medical Malpractice Exchange. It also provides news of case decisions, pleadings, and settlements in its periodical the *ATLA Law Reporter*.

The Environmental Law Institute offers case analyses and a litigation digest in its *Environmental Law Reporter* as well as a facsimile service for pleadings summarized in that periodical service. In addition, organizations such as the Environmental Defense Fund, the Natural Resources Defense Council, the Sierra Club, and the National Wildlife Federation have various legal projects related to toxic chemicals. These organizations have an interest in ensuring that the victims of toxic chemical pollutants are compensated for their damages. They are all involved, to some extent, in securing data from the federal government on toxics issues as well as in contributing to the federal regulatory decision-making process.

In addition, labor unions are also frequently involved with compensation issues and with developing epidemiologic data on occupational disease. Legal Services Corporation affiliates such as the Migrant Legal Action Program, Inc., and rural legal action organizations have also been active regarding toxic chemicals issues, particularly pesticides. Information on finding expert witnesses can be found under Health Effects (section 2) above.

Ecological Illness Law Report.

This 8-12 page newsletter, issued six times a year, addresses the legal problems generated for individuals who become ill or disabled owing to chemically induced immune disorders caused or triggered by chemicals in the workplace, home, or environment. Box 1739, Evanston, Illinois 60204.

Epstein, Samuel S. "The Role of the Scientist in Toxic Tort Case Preparation." *Trial* 17, no. 7 (July 1981): 38.

A very helpful discussion. *Trial* is published by the Association of Trial Lawyers of America, Washington, D.C.

Leape, James L. "Quantitative Risk Assessment in Regulation of Environmental Carcinogens." *Harvard Environmental Law Review* 4, no. 1 (1980): 86.

An excellent discussion of the development and use of regulatory risk assessment for environmental carcinogens. It discusses the legal implications of the various scientific techniques and protocols used in this process and makes recommendations on how risk assessments should be used in the regulatory process.

Page, Talbot. "A Generic View of Toxic Chemicals and Similar Risks." *Ecology Law Quarterly* 7, no. 2 (1978):207.

Discusses the nature of environmental risk and difficulties in managing it. Presents a theoretical view of the determination and evaluation of risks as well as methods of determining the "acceptability" of risks.

Toxic Torts: Tort Actions for Cancer and Lung Disease Due to Environmental Pollution. Washington, D.C.: Association of Trial Lawyers of America, 1977.

Includes chapters on the following topics: introduction to the toxic tort cause of action; chemical hazards—asbestos, vinyl chloride, PCBs, PBBs, kepone, dioxin, saccharin, Tris, radiation; law—information, Toxic Substances Control Act, nuisance, workers' compensation, nuclear accidents, overlooked occupational claims, OSHA, causation in environmental litigation, statutes of limitations.

Toxic Substances and Hazardous Wastes. ALI-ABA Course of Study Materials. Washington, D.C.: Environmental Law Institute, 1980.

Industrial and Toxic Torts. Washington, D.C.: 1980. Association of Trial Lawyers of America, 1980.

A guide to recognizing and handling personal injury cases arising from exposure to asbestos and radiation and from other chemical insults from toxic torts. Available for $45 ($35 to ATLA members) from Association of Trial Lawyers of America, Education Fund, P.O. box 3717, Georgetown, Washington, D.C. 20007, tel. (202) 965-3500.

Hazardous Substances in the Environment—Law and Policy. Special issue, *Ecology Law Quarterly* 7, no. 2 (1980):1-677.

This 677 page volume contains several important articles on the risks posed by toxic chemicals used in our society and how regulatory responses can be structured. Topics include a generic view of toxics risks, food and drugs, occupational health risks, international regulation, and a major case study of the ways the various federal agencies responded to the risks created by vinyl chloride. Available for $5 from School of Law, University of California, Berkeley, California 94720.

McGarity, Thomas O. "Finessing Causation: Three Novel Theories of Recovery for Carcinogenic Risk." In *Toxic Substances and Hazardous Wastes.* ALI-ABA Course of Study Materials. Washington, D.C.: Environmental Law Institute, 1980.

Six Case Studies of Compensation for Toxic Substances Pollution: Alabama, California, Michigan, Missouri, New Jersey, and Texas. Report prepared by the Congressional Research Service of the Library of Congress for the Committee on the Environment and Public Works, U.S. Senate, June 1980.

Doniger, David. *The Law and Policy of Toxic Substances Control: A Case Study of Vinyl Chloride.* Resources for the Future. Baltimore: Johns Hopkins University Press, 1978.

An Interim Report to Congress on Occupational Disease. Washington, D.C.: U.S. Department of Labor, 1980.

This report was requested by Congress in the Black Lung Benefits Reform Act of 1977 and is also referred to as the "Black Lung Benefits Act Study." It is an excellent summary of the effectiveness of various compensation systems for those who are victims of occupational diseases (rather than injuries) and is also applicable to the toxics compensation question in general.

Annual Committee Reports on Significant Legislative, Judicial, and Administrative Developments in 1979. Natural Resources Lawyer 13, nos. 1 and 2. Chicago: American Bar Association, 1980.

See the following sections:
Environmental Quality Committee, pp. 49–130.
Water Quality Committee, pp. 231–86.
Air Quality Committee, pp. 289–98.

Toxic Substances: Decisions and Values. Vol. 3. *Compensation.* Washington, D.C.: Technical Information Project, 1979.

This 90 page publication presents the basic issues in the compensation of victims of toxic substances pollution. It includes articles by Sheila Jasanoff and Stephen Soble, two leaders in this area. Available for $6 from Technical Information Project, 1346 Connecticut Avenue, NW, Suite 217, Washington, D.C. 20036.

Basic Science-Forcing Laws and Regulatory Case Studies: Kepone, DBCP, Halothane, Hexane and Carbaryl. Washington, D.C.: Environmental Law Institute, 1980.

McGarity, Thomas O. "Substantive and Procedural Discretion in Administrative Resolution of Science Policy Questions: Regulating Carcinogens in EPA and OSHA." *Georgetown Law Journal* 67:729.

Reprinted in *Toxic Substances and Hazardous Wastes.* ALI-ABA Course of Study Materials. Washington, D.C.: Environmental Law Institute, 1980.

Trauberman, Jeffrey, Durwood Zaelke, and Barbara Shaw. "The Citizen's Legal Guide to Hazardous Waste." In *Hazardous Waste in America,* ed. Samuel S. Epstein, Lester O. Brown, and Carl Pope. San Francisco: Sierra Club Books, 1982.

An excellent discussion of general legal theory and common law liability as applied to hazardous wastes, and a guide to what the citizen can do.

Trauberman, Jeffrey. "The Benzene Case: Adjudication on the Frontier of Science." In *Toxic Substances and Hazardous Wastes.* ALI-ABA Course of Study Materials. Washington, D.C.: Environmental Law Institute, 1980.

Canadian Law and the Control of Exposure to Hazards. Supply and Services of Canada (SSC110).

This 152 page book discusses legal aspects and issues relevant to the control and regulation of hazardous materials in Canada. The following are investigated: asbestos, lead, vinyl chloride monomer, mercury, oxides of nitrogen, and radiation. The book is available for $7.50 plus $1 postage and handling from UNIPUB, 345 Park Avenue South, New York, New York 10010.

Ewald, Thomas R. *Court Action for Migrants.* Washington, D.C.: Migrant Legal Action Program, 1972.

Skaff, Richard B. "The Emergency Powers in the Environmental Protection Statutes: A Suggestion for a Unified Emergency Provision." *Harvard Environmental Law Review* 3 (1979):298.

Farmworker Law: A Legal Service Practice Manual. Washington, D.C.: Migrant Legal Action Program, 1980.
Chapter 10, Occupational Safety and Health.
Chapter 11, Pesticides.

Bazelon, David L. "The Judiciary: What Role in Health Improvement?" *Science* 211 (20 February 1981):792–93.

Thomas, David B. "Lung Cancer and Ambient Air Pollution." *Environmental Law* 8, no. 3 (Spring 1978):701 (Lewis and Clark Law School, Northwestern School of Law).

Orloff, N., and Brooks, G. *The National Environmental Policy Act: Cases and Materials.* Washington, D.C.: Bureau of National Affairs, 1980.

This 532 page book is a broad introduction to the National Environmental Policy Act and the cases under it, as well as a comprehensive treatment of the Environmental Impact Statement process. Available for $25 from BNA Education Systems, Bureau of National Affairs, 9401 Decoverly Hall Road, Rockville, Maryland 20850.

Olpin, Owen. "Policing Toxic Chemicals." *Utah Law Review,* no. 1, 1976.
Available from University of Utah College of Law, Salt Lake City, Utah 84122.

Cottine, Bertram. "Public Health Decision-Making and the U.S. Legal Process: Regulation of Vinyl Chloride." *Annals of the New York Academy of Sciences* 329 (26 October 1979):188–200.

Friedman, Robert D. *Sensitive Populations and Environmental Standards: A Legal Analysis.* Washington, D.C.: Conservation Foundation, 1981.

This report, of approximately thirty-pages, addresses the issue of what population environmental standards are intended to protect and what problems arise because different people face different levels and types of risks from environmental pollutants. Available for $5 from The Conservation Foundation, 1717 Massachusetts Avenue, NW, Washington, D.C. 20036.

Bazelon, David L. "Science, Technology and the Court." *Science,* 208, no. 4445 (16 May 1980).

Futrell, J. William. "Toxic Substances, Environmental Mediation, and Lawyers." In *Toxic Substances and Hazardous Wastes.* ALI-ABA Course of Study Materials. Washington, D.C.: Environmental Law Institute, 1980.

"TSCA and Trade Secrets: Third Circuit Upholds EPA's Broad Authority to Obtain Health Studies under Section 8 (D)." *Environmental Law Reporter* 9 ELR (October 1979):10164.

McGarity, Thomas O., and Sidney A. Shapiro. "The Trade Secret Status of Health and Safety Testing Information: Reforming Agency Disclosure Policies." *Harvard Law Review* 93, no. 5 (March 1980):837–88.

Menottie, David. "Cost Sharing/Confidentiality: Problems with FIFRA and TSCA." In *Toxic Substances and Hazardous Wastes.* ALI-ABA Course of Study Materials. Washington, D.C.: Environmental Law Institute, 1980.

Grad, Frank, and Matthew Bender. *Treatise on Environmental Law.* 1980.

4. Epidemiology and Biostatistics

A. *Experts and Organizations*

Medical Schools and Public Health Schools

See the discussion under section 2.B above.

American Statistical Association
806 Fifteenth Street, NW, 6th Floor
Washington, D.C. 20005

Does not have a formal referral service, but does publish booklets and brochures, some written for the general public.

Society for Epidemiologic Research
c/o Dr. Susan T. Sacks, Epidemiology Division
University of California
School of Public Health
19 Earl Warren Hall
Berkeley, California 94720

National association of epidemiologists. Although it does not have a formal referral service, this professional organization could be useful in locating persons doing a specific type of research or an expert in a particular aspect of epidemiology.

B. *Publications*

Vital and Health Statistics. Washington, D.C.: Department of Health, Education, and Welfare.

An invaluable series of publications on collection procedures, data analysis, health surveys, special surveys, and other topics. Includes data from these surveys.

Mausner, Judith S., and Anita K. Bahn. *Epidemiology: An Introductory Text.* Philadelphia: W. B. Saunders, 1974.

Excellent 377 page text intended to provide a background in epidemiology. Discusses epidemiologic concepts and models, causal relations, types of epidemiologic studies, and sources of data on community health. Although written primarily for health workers, the style is clear and easily understood.

Friedman, Gary D. *Primer of Epidemiology.* New York: McGraw-Hill, 1980.

Good basic book on epidemiology.

Fisher, F. David. *An Introduction to Epidemiology: A Programmed Text.* New York: Appleton-Century-Crofts, 1975.

Self-teaching text of basic epidemiology. Frames 270-93, "General Review: Critiquing a Study," go through the major considerations in evaluating a journal article on a scientific study.

The Case of the Workplace Killers: A Manual for Cancer Detectives on the Job. Detroit: United Auto Workers, 1981.

This 40 page booklet describes ways workers can conduct studies to determine whether there is a higher risk of disease where they work. It also lists some high-risk UAW jobs and sources of additional information. Available for $1 from United Auto Workers, Purchase and Supply Department, 8000 E. Jefferson Street, Detroit, Michigan 48214.

Lave, Lester B., and Eugene P. Seskin. *Epidemiology, Causality, and Public Policy.* Reprint 165. Resources for the Future. Baltimore: Johns Hopkins University Press, 1979.

Ferfer, Robert, Paul Sheatsley, Anthony Turner, and Joseph Waksberg. *What Is a Survey?* Washington, D.C.: American Statistical Association, 1980.

This 25 page booklet looks at what is involved in carrying out a sample survey and lists aspects that need to be considered to evaluate the results. Written for those with no formal training in statistics.

Tanur, Janet, et al. *Statistics: A Guide to the Unknown.* San Francisco: Holden-Day, 1972.

Book on survey methods written for nontechnical readers.

Hauser, Philip. *Social Statistics in Use.* New York: Russell Sage Foundation, 1975.

Another book on survey methods written for the nonstatistician.

Williams, William H. *A Sampler on Sampling.* New York: John Wiley, 1978.

Written for the nonstatistician.

Statistics Needed for Determining the Effects of the Environment on Health: Report of the Technical Consultant Panel to the U.S. National Committee on Vital and Health Statistics. Health Resources Administration Series 4, no. 20. Washington, D.C.: U.S. Department of Health, Education, and Welfare, Public Health Service, 1977.

Fox, John P., Carrie Hall, and Lila R. Elveback. "Disease Causation: General Concepts and the Nature and Classification of Disease Agents." In *Epidemiology: Man and Disease,* chap. 3. London: Macmillan, 1970.

Discusses the contributing factors that must be analyzed when evaluating causation. These contributing factors or secondary causes influence disease occurrence in important ways, even when the primary cause is known. Chapters cover primary cause and contributing factors, classes of contributing factors and their interaction, and nature and classification of disease agents.

Susser, Mervyn. "Procedures for Establishing Causal Association." In *Trends in Epidemiology: Application to Health Service Research and Training,* ed. Gordon T. Stewart, chap. 2. Springfield, Ill.: Charles C. Thomas, 1972.

This 80 page chapter on how to "prove" causation reviews the types of associations and a number of strategies for dispelling false inferences. Research design and statistical approaches are briefly discussed; the search for extraneous sources of variation that can produce observed associations between variables, the elaboration of the analysis of associated variables, and criteria of judgment are treated at greater length.

Susser, Mervyn. *Causal Thinking in the Health Sciences: Concepts and Strategies of Epidemiology.* New York: Oxford University Press, 1973.

Expansion of Susser's chapter "Procedures for Establishing Causal Associations," listed above.

MacMahon, Brian, and Thomas F. Pugh. "Concepts of Cause." In *Epidemiology: Principles and Methods,* chap. 2. Boston: Little, Brown, 1970.

Discusses the types of association, some criteria for distinguishing between causal and noncausal association, direct and indirect association, the "web of causation," and causation and prevention.

Lilienfeld, Abraham M. "Derivation of Etiological Hypotheses from Epidemiological Studies." In *Foundations of Epidemiology,* chap 12. New York: Oxford University Press, 1976.

Deals with the explanatory hypotheses that can be inferred once a pattern of statistical relations has been observed between a disease and biological or social characteristics. Draws mainly on data from studies of cigarette smoking and lung cancer to illustrate major principles.

Hill, Austin Bradford. "The Environment and Disease: Association or Causation?" *Proceedings of the Royal Society of Medicine* (1965):295–300.

Rothman, Kenneth J. "Causes." *American Journal of Epidemiology* 104, no. 6 (December 1976): 587–92.

Clarifies the concept of multicausality by noting that causes in and of themselves are rarely sufficient to produce a single effect. The concepts of component and sufficient causes are discussed.

Koopman, James S. "Causal Models and Sources of Interaction." *American Journal of Epidemiology* 106, no. 6 (December 1977):439–44.

Cochran, William G. "The Role of Statistics in National Health Policy Decisions." *American Journal of Epidemiology* 104, no. 4 (1976): 370–85.

Discusses the role of the statistician in national health policy decisions. Considers the two major branches of methodological statistics: sample surveys and techniques for studying the effects of different procedures or agents. Discusses issues that arise in using these techniques as a guide for health policy decisions, such as preparing summaries of the state of the evidence and monitoring and evaluating policies in operation.

Ipsen, Johannes, and Polly Feigl. *Introduction to Biostatistics.* 2d ed. New York: Harper and Row, 1970.

Textbook for health-science students. Chapter 16, "Design of Experiment," deals with such issues as systematic error, sample size, precision, and statistical design.

England, John M. *Medical Research.* New York: Churchill Livingstone, 1975.

Chapter 1, An Introduction to the Important Terminology; chapter 3, Planning an Investigation; chapter 4, How Many Subjects Need to Be Studied; a chapter on analyzing results. Chapter 12 gives a brief synopsis of how to read a scientific article ("Hints on Reading a Publication"). Straightforward language, intermediate level.

Leaver, R. H., and T. R. Thomas. *Analysis and Presentation of Experimental Results.* New York: John Wiley, 1974.

An advanced text on statistical analysis. Pages xi–xiii show "flow charts for error analysis" that outline the various statistical analyses and tell when they should be used. Chapter citations are given there so that the reader can then refer to the appropriate chapters.

Journals

American Journal of Epidemiology
Journal of the American Statistical Association
American Statistician

5. Risk Assessment

Leape, James L. "Quantitative Risk Assessment in Regulation of Environmental Carcinogens." *Harvard Environmental Law Review* 4, no. 1 (1980): 86.

An excellent discussion of the development and use of regulatory risk assessments for environmental carcinogens. It discusses the legal implications of the various scientific techniques and protocols used in this process and presents recommendations on how risk assessments should be used in the regulatory process.

Page, Talbot. "A Generic View of Toxic Chemicals and Similar Risks." *Ecology Law Quarterly* 7, no. 2 (1978):207.

Discusses the nature of environmental risk and difficulties in managing it. It presents a theoretical view of the determination and evaluation of risks as well as methods of determining the "acceptability" of risks.

Davis, D. L. and D. P. Rall. "Risk Assessment for Disease Prevention." In *Strategies for Public Health,* ed. L. K. Y. Ng and D. L. Davis, chap. 9. New York: Van Nostrand Reinhold, 1981.

Davis, Devra Lee. "Multiple Risk Assessment: Preventive Strategy for Public Health." *Toxic Substances Journal* 1 (1979):205.

Davies, J. C., S. Gusman, and F. Irwin. "Determining Unreasonable Risk." In *Strategies for Public Health,* ed. L. K. Y. Ng and D. L. Davis, chap. 12. New York: Van Nostrand Reinhold, 1981.

"Environmental Health Issues" (Risk assessment; How does science assess hazards of chemicals to humans? . . .). *Environmental Science and Technology* 15, no. 3 (March 1981):248–49.

Kamlet, Kenneth S. "Federal Environmental Legislation: Problems of Risk Assessment and Standard Setting." In *Toxic Substances and Hazardous Wastes.* ALI-ABA Course of Study Materials. Washington, D.C.: Environmental Law Institute, 1980.

"National Institute on Law, Science and Technology in Health Risk Regulation." Special issue of *Jurimetrics Journal* vol. 19, no. 5 (1980). American Bar Association.

Humpstone, Charles C. "Pollution Insurance Comes of Age." *Risk Management,* August 1977.

Pollution's "Invisible" Victims: Why Environmental Regulation Cannot Wait for Scientific Certainty. EPA OPA119/0. Washington, D.C.: U.S. Environmental Protection Agency, 1980.

Throdahl, Monte C. "Risk Management as Self-Discipline." *Technology Review,* October 1980, p. 12.

Bazelon, David L. "Risk and Responsibility." *Science* 205 (20 July 1979): 277–80.

"The Risky Business of Assessing Risk." *Environmental Science and Technology* 14, no. 11 (November 1980):1281–82.

Brady, Gordon L. and Blair T. Bower. "Benefit-Cost Analysis in Air Quality Management." *Environmental Science and Technology* 15, no. 3 (March 1981):257.

Freeman, A. Myrick, III. *The Benefits of Environmental Improvement.* Resources for the Future. Baltimore: Johns Hopkins University Press, 1979.

Chapters include discussions of benefit measures from the following perspectives: limitations of measurements and attributing values by market and nonmarket means, property values, longevity, recreation, and productivity.

"Counting All the Costs: Science and Judgment in Chemical Control." Remarks made by Russell W. Peterson, chairman, Council on Environmental Quality, 16 March 1976. Society of Toxicology Annual Meeting, Marriott Hotel, Atlanta, Georgia.

Cost Benefit Analysis and Environmental, Health and Safety Regulation: An Overview of the Agencies and Legislation. Washington, D.C.: Environmental Law Institute, Toxic Substances Program, 1980.

"Cost-Benefit Analysis." *Environmental Science and Technology* 14, no. 12 (December 1980):1415.

The Economy and the Environment. EPA Journal Reprint OPA59/9. Washington, D.C.: U.S. Environmental Protection Agency, 1979.

Saving Ourselves Broke: The Future Expenses of Deferred Regulation. OPA75/9. Washington, D.C.: U.S. Environmental Protection Agency, 1979.

This EPA pamphlet discusses the future costs we will have to pay if we are shortsighted in the present and fail to take effective action in controlling pollutants.

Journals

Regulatory Toxicology and Pharmacology

Relates scientific and legal concepts concerning human health and the environment. It reports ideas and propositions developed in the writing and speeches of lawyers, scientists, business people, the public, and government officials.

6. Directories, Guides, and Catalogues

Contact: Toxics—a Guide to Specialists on Toxic Substances. New York: World Environment Center.

Lists the names, telephone numbers, and professional profiles of almost a thousand specialists involved in the manufacture, handling, and disposal of toxic substances. Available for $37.50 for nonprofit organizations ($49.50 for government and industry) from World Environment Center, 300 East 42d Street, New York, New York 10017, tel. (212) 697-3232. WEC also publishes a newsletter called the *World Environment Report.*

Experts List. Washington, D.C.: Environmental Action Foundation, Waste and Toxic Substances Project, 1981.

Information on experts available to assist and advise citizens in the areas related to toxic substances, maintained on a referral service basis by this organization. For more information call (202) 296-7570 or write to Waste and Toxic Substances Project, Environmental Action Foundation, 724 Dupont Circle Building, Washington, D.C. 20036.

Toxic Substances Sourcebook II. New York: Environment Information Center, 1980.

Comprehensive 550 page guide to information sources, key literature, and laws on toxic substances. Available for $95 from Environment Information Center, 292 Madison Avenue, New York, New York 10017.

Waste Alert. Washington, D.C.: Technical Information Project, 1981.

This newsletter is part of the Waste Alert Project sponsored by the Environmental Protection Agency and developed by the League of Women Voters Education Fund, the American Public Health Association, the Environmental Action Foundation, the Izaak Walton League of America, the National Wildlife Federation, and the Technical Information Project. Available from Technical Information Project, 1346 Connecticut Avenue, NW, Suite 217, Washington, D.C. 20036.

Water Quality Management Directory. 3d ed. Washington, D.C.: U.S. Environmental Protection Agency, 1979.

World Environmental Directory. Silver Spring, Md.: Business Publishers, 1980.

This 1,088 page directory lists environmental equipment manufacturers, consultants, regulatory personnel in government and industry, environmental attorneys, university programs, professional and scientific societies, libraries, periodicals, and more. Available for $67.50 from Business Publishers, P.O. box 1067, Silver Spring, Maryland 10910, tel. (301) 587-6300.

Pollution Equipment News. Pittsburgh, Pa.: Richard Rimbauch, 1968-.

This extensive catalog of environmental pollution detection and control equipment and services is available free. For a subscription write to Pollution Equipment News, Circulation Office, 8650 Babcock Boulevard, Pittsburgh, Pennsylvania 15237.

Catalogue (1981-GB General Catalogue). Tempe, Ariz.: Direct Safety Company, 1981.

This safety equipment catalog may be obtained from Direct Safety Company, 1607 W. 17th Street, P.O. Box 26616, Tempe, Arizona 85282.

Catalogue, Industrial Safety Products. Rockford, Ill. Rockford Safety Equipment Company, 1980.

Copies may be obtained from Rockford Safety Equipment Company, 4620 Hydraulic Road, P.O. box 5166, Rockford, Illinois 61125.

1981 Catalogue and Buyer's Guide. Pittsburgh, Pa.: Richard Rimbauch, 1980.

A product and manufacturer directory for pollution control, detection, and safety equipment and services. It may be obtained from the same address as *Pollution Equipment News,* listed above.

Topical Directory. A-107, OPA 120/9. Washington, D.C.: U.S. Environmental Protection Agency, Office of Public Awareness, 1980.

Arranged by substantive areas rather than by programs and divisions. For each area of research or program activities, one person is identified as the primary contact, and a telephone number is given. Although many entries are out of date, this is still an invaluable guide to EPA activities.

Conservation Directory 1981. 26th ed. Washington, D.C.: National Wildlife Federation, 1981.

This comprehensive annual directory, listing major national and local private organizations as well as government offices, is available for $6 from The National Wildlife Federation, 1412 Sixteenth Street, NW, Washington, D.C. 20036, tel. (202) 797-6800.

A Guide to Worker Education Materials in Occupational Safety and Health. Washington, D.C.: Occupational Safety and Health Administration, 1979.

Prepared by Urban Environment Conference. See next entry for availability.

A Guide to Worker Education Materials in Occupational Safety and Health. Vol. 2. Washington, D.C.: Occupational Safety and Health Administration, 1980.

Prepared by the Urban Environment Conference. Available from U.S. Department of Labor—OSHA, Office of Publication Distribution, Room S-1212, Third and Constitution Avenue, NW, Washington, D.C. 20210.

Chemical Regulation Reporter. Washington, D.C.: Bureau of National Affairs, 1981.

This multivolume, constantly updated binder series includes the following coverages of chemical regulations in every government arena:
Current Reports—A weekly magazine, indexed.

Reference File—Compilation of all laws and regulations related to chemical products.

Hazardous Materials Transportation—An easy reference guide to the provisions of the Hazardous Materials Transportation Act.

Index to Government Regulations.

This service is available from the Bureau of National Affairs, 1231 Twenty-fifth Street, NW, Washington, D.C. 20037

Directory of Federal Coordinating Groups for Toxic Substances. 2d ed. Toxics Integration Information Series, EPA-560/13-80-008. Washington, D.C.: U.S. Environmental Protection Agency, Office of Pesticides and Toxic Substances, 1980.

Available from the Industry Assistance Office at EPA, tel. toll free (800) 424-9065, or call (202) 554-1404.

Directory of Federal Interagency Groups Concerned with Environmental Health. Washington, D.C.: U.S. Task Force on Environmental Cancer and Heart and Lung Disease, 1979.

This task force includes the following members: Environmental Protection Agency, National Cancer Institute, National Heart, Lung, and Blood Institute, National Institute for Occupational Safety and Health, National Institute of Environmental Health Science, National Center for Health Statistics, Center for Disease Control, and Food and Drug Administration.

Environmental Glossary. Washington, D.C.: Government Institutes, 1980.

This glossary contains over two thousand terms, abbreviations, and acronyms, all compiled directly from the environmental statutes, the Code of Federal Regulations, or the EPA. It is available for approximately $20 from Government Institutes, P.O. box 5918, Washington, D.C. 20014, tel. (301) 656-1090 (Rockville, Maryland).

Environment Information Center (information services).

Environment Abstracts—Monthly abstracts of articles from environmental publications.

Environment Index—Index to documents in *Environment Abstracts* plus directory information.

Environment Abstracts Annual—Cumulative edition of *Environment Abstracts.*

Environment Regulation Handbook—Covers all environmental laws and regulations.

Available from Environment Information Center, 292 Madison Avenue, New York, New York, 10017, tel. (212) 949-9494.

Publications on Toxic Substances: A Descriptive Listing. Washington, D.C.: Interagency Regulatory Liaison Group, 1979.

Publications, Environmental Law Institute

ELI has several excellent publications on toxic chemicals and other environmental law concerns. The publications list may be ordered from Publications, Environmental Law Institute, 1346 Connecticut Avenue, NW, Washington, D.C. 20036, tel. (202) 452-9600.

Natural Resources Defense Council: Current Publications List. New York: Natural Resources Defense Council, 1980.

This list contains NRDC publications on air, coastal zone management, energy, forestry, international pollution, land use, toxic substances/health, transportation, wildlife, litigation, and other environmental considerations. The list and publications can be ordered from Publications Office, Natural Resources Defense Council, 122 East 42d Street, New York, New York, 10017, tel. (212) 949-0049.

Resource Guide: Waste and Toxic Substances. Washington, D.C.: Environmental Action Foundation, 1981.

This 30 page pamphlet lists resource materials in the following areas: general solid waste, waste reduction and conservation of materials, environmental education, media, citizen organizing, hazardous wastes, toxic substances, and occupational environmental health and safety. *Environmental Action* magazine reprints, environmental films, and other materials are included. Available for $1 from Environmental Action Foundation, Waste and Toxic Substances Project, 724 Dupont Circle Building, Washington, D.C. 20036, tel. (202) 296-7570.

Publications List. Washington, D.C.: Environmental Defense Fund, Toxic Chemicals Program, 1980.

Publications include reports, comments, petitions, pleadings, and so on, prepared by EDF's Toxic Chemical Program. The 33 page list is available from Publications, Environmental Defense Fund, 1525 Eighteenth Street, NW, Washington, D.C. 20036, tel. (202) 883-1484.

Appendix
Rates of Cancer
and Birth Defects

We have stressed throughout this manual that it is imperative to survey an unexposed or control population in exactly the same manner and with the same care as you survey your own community. As a poor second choice, we are providing some national rates or sources of such information, with all the drawbacks inherent in such figures.

Most of the symptoms or conditions uncovered by a community health survey will be acute, temporary, or subclinical. Generally speaking, there is almost no information on these kinds of conditions other than rough guesses published by national associations (professional or lay) for particular diseases, or by insurance companies who have to pay for much of the associated medical care, or as results of large health surveys (HANES [Second National Health and Nutrition Examination Survey, a survey of adults conducted by the Public Health Service], Framingham, and others) to which professionals or officials should have access. A few serious diseases must be reported to the Centers for Disease Control. These "notifiable" diseases include aseptic meningitis, encephalitis (primary and postinfectious), gonorrhea, hepatitis, Legionellosis, leprosy, malaria, measles, meningococcic infections, mumps, pertussis, rubella (German measles), syphilis, toxic shock syndrome, tuberculosis, tularemia, typhoid fever, typhus, rabies, and some low-frequency illnesses (plague, polio, anthrax, tetanus, etc.).

Some information is available from the Public Health Service concerning health care use (how many times people see a doctor, how long they are hospitalized, what operations they have, and so on). Most of the rates calculated from these studies concern the major fatal diseases. Inquiries can be addressed to U.S. Department of Health and Human Services, Public Health Service, Office of Health Research, Statistics, and Technology, or Office of Disease Prevention and Health Promotion, National Center for Health Statistics, 3700 East West Highway, Hyattsville, Maryland 20782, tel. (301) 436–6247.

A sample of publications from the Public Health service includes: *Vital and Health Statistics* (a serial available from libraries at many medical schools or schools of public health), "Health United States, 1980" (DHHS Publication [PHS] 81–1232), and "Prevention '80" (DHHS Publication [PHS] 81–50157).

National averages of leading causes of death give some information on major health conditions, and presumably each patient has had a disease for a while before dying from it (table A.1). However, these and the following rates (tables A.2–A.4) include only patients who die, whereas community health surveys are concerned almost entirely with health before death. Note that the same source, National Center for Health Statistics (NCHS), lists the total death rate for 1978 both as 883 per 100,000 (table A.3) and as 606 per 100,000 (table A.4).

These same rates from NCHS (*Vital and Health Statistics,* 1978) are cited by other sources (American Cancer Society, for example), as different yet (table A.5).

This should give you an idea of the accuracy of such rates. On the whole, published cancer rates average from 17 or 18 percent to 22 or 23 percent of all causes of death. Another problem in comparing death rates is that, for instance for cardiovascular diseases, it is not clear whether ischemic heart disease includes atherosclerosis and angina as well as heart attacks, whether cerebrovascular disease includes both cerebral hemorrhage and cerebral thrombosis, whether arteriosclerosis and hypertension are included under the umbrella of major cardiovascular disease, and so on.

Cancer statistics have also been widely published. Probably the most accurate rates were determined by the National Cancer Institute as part of the SEER (Surveillance and Epidemiology End

Results) reports. They are published as S. J. Cutler and J. L. Young, eds., *Third National Cancer Survey: Incidence Data,* National Cancer Institute Monograph 41, DHEW no. (NIH) 75-787 (Bethesda, Md.: National Cancer Institute, Biometry Branch, Division of Cancer Cause and Prevention, 1975). This publication can be obtained from U.S. Department of Health and Human Services, Public Health Service, National Institutes of Health, National Cancer Institute, Bethesda, Maryland 20014. These rates were determined from seven metropolitan areas plus two entire states, based on deaths occurring from 1969 to 1971. The total population of these areas was 21,003,451, out of a total United States population of 203,211,926. Close to 10 percent of the total United States population was surveyed, each race was included, and the age distribution closely matched the national pattern. Most (90 percent) of the cancer cases were confirmed either by cytological evaluation or by hospital records (tables A.6–A.8). In this publication the overall crude mortality rate of all cancer per 100,000 population is given as 287, much higher than the National Center for Health Statistics calculation for 1978.

The American Cancer Society also publishes annual cancer statistics, and these figures vary greatly from the National Cancer Institute for particular sites. One can see how the controversy arises concerning whether cancer rates are increasing or decreasing. Is the two-year or five-year survival a "cure"? Are these rates calculated from "new cases" or from "deaths"? Does postponing death by effective treatment mean that future rates will rise? Have all cancer cases been reported and all cancer deaths accurately recorded?

It should be apparent that a single national average for a particular condition or cancer site will not be very useful for purposes of a community health survey. The first point to remember is that cancer rates in general increase with age (table A.9, fig. A.1). The second point is that some cancers have peak incidence rates at different ages (leukemia peaks in childhood, then again in old age). Therefore rates for each group are needed for comparisons.

Another factor that must be taken into account is the geographic distributions both of some malignant and of some non-malignant conditions. The most striking example of this is ischemic heart disease, with rates taken from Mason et al. (1975a; cited by W. Villanueva in *Discover* magazine, September 1982, p. 82). The east/west variation makes it clear that a national incidence rate might not be at all comparable to the rate in your community. The best example of a population-based tumor registry is the Connecticut Tumor Registry, Connecticut State Department of Health, Hartford, Connecticut.

There are many other examples of geographic differences: intestinal infectious disease is more common in the Southwest; tuberculosis is more common in Appalachia and southern Texas and among American Indians; multiple sclerosis shows a north/south gradient. These statistics, while they can be used for illustration, lack some precision because the information comes from death certificates from 1965–71, based on a 1960 census population and extrapolated to later years, and some information comes from death certificates in rural areas where there might have been no medically trained coroner or medical examiner (fig. A.2).

The third type of national rates you might need are for birth defects or congenital malformations. In general these rates are more accurate because each case must be reported when recognized, and most conditions are fairly easy for a trained pediatrician to recognize. Again, there are some geographic gradients, especially for spina bifida and hip dislocation, as reported by the Centers for Disease Control (1980) in congenital malformations surveillance reports. For comparison, rates from Bloom (1981) are given for congenital anomalies seen in over 30,000 births at the Boston Hospital for Women. Some rates show more than a twofold difference from the Centers for Disease Control figures, for which we currently have no explanation. In addition, minor anomalies may escape notice during the first year and thus be underreported (table A.10).

In conclusion, discrepancies in incidence and mortality rates collected by various groups and widely quoted or misquoted demonstrate the difficulty of accurately measuring background rates of major diseases or conditions. However, for rare conditions they may be the only information available, in which case we must choose what appears to be the most accurate data set to use in calculating how many cases would be expected in a smaller population. For acute or less serious conditions, there is very little reliable (quantitative) information upon which either you or state health officials can base calculations, so there is no alternative to collecting it yourself.

Table A.1 Death Rates from Specified Causes, by Race and Sex: United States, 1978 (per 100,000)

Cause of Death	Total			White			All Other Races		
	Both Sexes	Male	Female	Both Sexes	Male	Female	Both Sexes	Male	Female
All causes	883.4	994.4	778.3	895.7	999.8	796.5	805.1	959.7	664.5
Major cardiovascular diseases	442.7	472.8	414.2	459.5	489.2	431.2	335.5	365.6	308.1
Diseases of heart	334.3	375.3	295.5	348.6	390.8	308.4	204.8	273.8	214.7
Hypertension	2.5	2.4	2.6	2.3	2.2	2.4	3.7	3.8	3.6
Cerebrovascular diseases	10.4	9.6	20.3	18.4	15.3	21.4	13.5	13.2	13.7
Arteriosclerosis	13.3	10.9	9.7	12.8	15.7	10.1	8.0	8.7	7.3
Cancer	181.9	203.5	161.4	186.6	206.4	167.7	152.0	184.9	122.1
Accidents	48.4	69.6	28.3	47.9	68.3	28.5	51.3	78.2	26.8
Motor vehicle accidents	24.0	35.9	12.7	24.4	36.2	13.1	21.8	34.1	10.6
All other accidents	24.4	33.7	15.5	23.5	32.1	15.4	29.5	44.1	16.3
Influenza and pneumonia	1.9	1.6	2.1	2.0	1.7	2.3	0.9	0.9	0.9
Cirrhosis of the liver	13.8	18.6	9.3	13.2	17.8	8.8	17.5	23.3	12.3
Diabetes mellitus	15.5	13.1	17.8	15.0	12.9	17.0	18.7	14.7	22.5
Suicide	12.5	19.0	6.3	13.4	20.2	6.9	6.9	11.1	3.1
Homocide	9.4	14.9	4.1	5.9	9.2	2.9	31.2	52.6	11.8
Bronchitis, emphysema, and asthma	10.0	14.4	5.9	10.8	15.5	6.4	5.0	7.3	2.9
Tuberculosis, all forms	1.3	1.8	0.9	1.1	1.4	0.7	3.0	4.3	1.7

Source: National Center for Health Statistics. Cited in *Hammond Almanac* (1983).

Table A.2 Death Rates for Various Age Groups, by Race and Sex: United States, 1978 (per 100,000)

Age Group	Total			White			All Other Races		
	Both Sexes	Male	Female	Both Sexes	Male	Female	Both Sexes	Male	Female
All ages[a]	883.4	994.4	778.3	895.7	999.8	796.5	805.1	959.7	664.5
Under 1 year	1,434.4	1,591.7	1,269.6	1,218.3	1,359.6	1,069.7	2,456.7	2,798.5	2,206.5
1–4	69.2	78.1	59.9	62.7	71.7	53.3	99.0	108.1	89.7
5–9	33.4	38.9	27.8	31.4	36.3	26.3	43.0	51.5	34.4
10–14	34.3	43.7	24.6	33.0	41.8	23.7	40.9	53.1	28.6
15–19	100.9	145.3	55.3	101.8	146.9	55.2	96.0	136.1	55.9
20–24	134.7	203.1	66.5	126.3	190.8	61.0	184.0	278.4	97.2
25–29	131.8	192.2	72.5	115.7	168.3	63.0	233.7	356.7	128.5
30–34	139.7	192.9	87.8	120.6	165.0	76.4	270.5	402.3	159.7
35–39	189.4	254.0	127.9	161.7	215.3	109.6	381.6	548.8	244.8
40–44	296.1	382.8	213.8	257.2	329.1	187.5	562.6	784.7	380.9
45–49	471.6	608.5	341.4	428.5	553.8	307.8	779.7	1,021.3	570.1
50–54	742.4	980.9	520.5	683.7	906.6	474.5	1,216.8	1,610.3	877.4
55–59	1,115.9	1,490.1	774.3	1,046.0	1,404.8	716.5	1,734.2	2,266.7	1,271.5
60–64	1,774.2	2,411.5	1,212.8	1,695.2	2,318.2	1,143.4	2,537.7	3,339.1	1,867.3
65–69	2,463.0	3,439.3	1,685.2	2,412.7	3,394.5	1,628.2	2,878.3	3,814.8	2,150.3
70–74	3,787.4	5,241.5	2,724.9	3,684.9	5,166.9	2,612.5	4,877.9	5,984.5	3,980.1
75–79	6,024.2	8,065.8	4,713.2	5,393.8	7,996.2	4,564.3	7,547.7	8,724.1	6,620.7
80–84	8,954.0	11,597.1	7,509.4	9,080.7	11,821.8	7,606.7	7,573.2	9,419.8	6,372.9
85 and over	14,700.7	17,258.9	13,541.2	15,316.0	18,100.3	14,079.0	9,228.7	10,678.2	8,449.0

Source: National Center for Health Statistics. Cited in *Hammond Almanac* (1983).

[a]Figures for age not stated are included in "all ages" but not distributed among age groups.

Table A.3   Leading Causes of Death in the United States, 1978

Rank	Cause of Death	Number of Deaths	Death Rate per 100,000
	All Causes	1,927,788	883.4
1	Heart diseases	729,510	334.3
2	Cancer	396,992	181.9
3	Cerebrovascular diseases	175,629	80.5
4	Accidents	105,561	48.4
	Motor vehicle accidents	52,411	24.0
	All other	53,150	24.4
5	Influenza and pneumonia	58,319	26.7
6	Diabetes mellitus	33,841	15.5
7	Cirrhosis of the liver	30,066	13.8
8	Arteriosclerosis	28,940	13.3
9	Suicide	27,294	12.5
10	Diseases of early infancy	22,033	10.1
	All other causes	319,603	146.5

Source: National Center for Health Statistics. Cited in *Hammond Almanac* (1983).

Table A.4   Leading Causes of Death in the United States, 1978

Cause of Death	Percentage of Total Deaths	Death Rate per 100,000
All causes	100.0	606
Heart disease	34.3	208
Cancer	22.1	134
Stroke	7.5	45
Accidents	7.3	44
Influenza and pneumonia	2.5	15
Suicide	2.0	12
Diabetes mellitus	1.7	10

Source: National Center for Health Statistics, "Final Mortality Statistics, 1978," *Monthly Vital Statistics Report,* vol. 29, no. 6, suppl. 2, 17 September 1980.

Table A.5   Leading Causes of Death in the United States, 1978

Cause of Death	Percentage of Total Deaths	Death Rate per 100,000
All causes	100.0	810.0
Heart disease	37.8	300.4
Cancer	20.6	169.9
Cerebrovascular diseases	9.1	70.8
Accidents	5.5	45.8
Pneumonia and influenza	3.0	23.6
Chronic obstructive lung diseases	2.6	21.2
Diabetes mellitus	1.8	14.2
Cirrhosis of the liver	1.6	13.4
Arteriosclerosis	1.5	11.1
Suicide	1.4	11.6
Diseases of infancy	1.1	12.1
Homicide	1.1	8.7
Aortic aneurysm	0.8	5.8
Congenital anomalies	0.7	6.8
Pulmonary infarction	0.6	4.6
Other and ill defined	10.8	89.9

Source: National Center for Health Statistics, *Vital Statistics of the United States,* 1978, as cited by the American Cancer Society, *Cancer Statistics,* vol. 33, no. 1, 1983.

Table A.6   Percentage of Cancer Mortality by Primary Site, Not Divided by Race, Sex, and Area, out of 181,027 Cases, 1969–71

Site or Type of Cancer	Percentage
All sites	100
Mouth and pharynx	3.6
Digestive system	25.1
	(10.2 of which is colon cancer)
Respiratory system	15.0
Bones and joints	0.3
Soft tissue	0.7
Skin (melanomas)	1.4
Breast	13.6
Female genitals	10.3
	(20.6 of female cancers)
Male genitals	8.9
	(20.6 of male cancers)
Urinary tract	6.6
Brain and nervous system	1.7
Endocrine system	1.4
Eye and orbit	0.3
Lymphoma	3.3
Multiple myeloma	1.2
Leukemia	3.3
Unknown	3.5

Source: Mason et al. (1975a), Third National Cancer Survey, Surveillance and Epidemiology End Results (SEER) Program, National Cancer Institute.

Table A.7   Estimated Cancer Incidence by Site and Sex, 1983

Site or Type of Cancer	Percentage of All Cancer Cases	
	Male	Female
All sites	100	100
Skin	2	2
Mouth and pharynx	4	2
Lung	22	9
Breast	—	26
Pancreas	3	3
Colon and rectum	14	15
Prostate	18	—
Urinary tract	9	4
Ovary	—	4
Uterus	—	13
Leukemia and lymphomas	8	7
All other	20	15

Source: SEER program, National Cancer Institute, cited by the American Cancer Institute, cited by the American Cancer Society in *Ca-A Cancer Journal for Clinicians,* vol. 33, no. 1, 1983.

Table A.8   Estimated Cancer Deaths by Site and Sex, 1983

Site or Type of Cancer	Percentage of All Cancer Deaths	
	Male	Female
All sites	100	100
Skin	2	1
Mouth and pharynx	3	1
Lung	35	17
Breast	—	18
Pancreas	5	5
Colon and rectum	12	15
Prostate	10	—
Urinary tract	5	3
Ovary	—	6
Uterus	—	5
Leukemia and lymphomas	8	9
All other	20	20

Source: National Cancer Institute, SEER program, cited by the American Cancer Society.

Table A.9   Age-Specific Rates of Cancer, United States
            Whites, 1950–69 (per 100,000)

Age	Males	Females
0–4	11.27	9.66
5–9	9.07	7.04
10–14	6.75	5.35
15–19	9.34	6.12
20–24	11.25	7.39
25–29	14.52	12.75
30–34	20.72	25.39
35–39	33.60	48.72
40–44	62.09	89.30
45–49	116.16	144.60
50–54	214.16	214.00
55–59	358.95	292.52
60–64	559.46	387.33
65–69	787.99	505.30
70–74	1,052.62	663.23
75–84	1,454.51	935.09
85+	1,798.98	1,231.15

Source: Mason et al. (1975a).

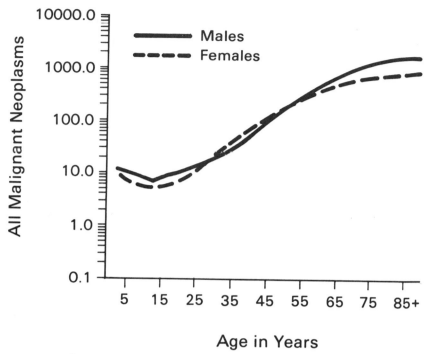

Figure A.1   Age-Specific Rates of Cancer
Source: Mason et al. 1975.

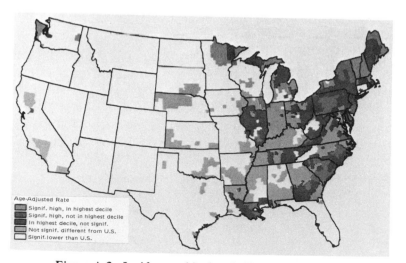

Figure A.2   Incidence of Ischemic Heart Disease

Table A.10 Incidence of Selected Congenital Malformations per 10,000 Births

Malformation	Northeast	North Central	South	West	Total United States
Central nervous system					
Anencephaly					
1970–73	5.1	4.9	5.8	5.1	5.2
1979	3.3	3.9	3.5	3.3	3.6
1980	3.7	3.1	3.8	2.5	3.3
Spina bifida without anencephaly					
1970–73	6.9	7.1	8.7	5.6	7.2
1979	5.1	5.1	5.1	4.4	5.0
1980	3.8	5.1	6.9	4.0	5.2
Hydrocephalus without spina bifida					
1970–73	4.7	4.8	5.0	4.2	4.7
1979	4.8	4.6	4.7	4.0	4.6
1980	3.9	3.9	4.6	3.4	4.0
Cardiovascular					
Transposition of great vessels					
1970–73	0.9	0.8	0.7	0.9	0.8
1979	1.1	1.1	0.8	1.2	1.0
1980	0.9	0.7	0.8	0.5	0.7
Ventricular septal defect					
1970–73	5.8	4.6	4.5	7.1	5.2
1979	12.2	10.7	8.6	12.5	10.7
1980	14.5	11.3	10.3	12.4	11.7
Patent ductus arteriosus					
1970–73	4.6	4.6	4.3	8.5	5.1
1979	16.8	17.9	13.7	19.7	16.8
1980	17.1	15.8	16.1	19.2	16.7
Craniofacial					
Cleft palate without cleft lip					
1970–73	5.7	5.4	4.7	5.6	5.3
1979	4.3	5.7	5.2	4.9	5.2
1980	3.9	5.2	4.6	5.4	4.9
Cleft lip with or without cleft palate					
1970–73	9.2	10.6	9.2	11.2	10.0
1979	5.7	8.6	7.7	7.8	7.7
1980	6.6	8.4	7.7	8.9	8.0
Musculoskeletal					
Clubfoot without CNS anomalies					
1970–73	33.6	33.5	21.5	23.1	29.4
1979	30.8	28.7	20.1	20.9	25.3
1980	30.2	29.8	21.5	18.7	25.7

Table A.10 (continued)

Malformation	Northeast	North Central	South	West	Total United States
Reduction deformity					
1970–73	2.9	3.0	3.1	4.0	3.1
1979	3.6	3.7	3.1	4.0	3.6
1980	4.4	3.9	3.4	3.8	3.8
Hip dislocation without CNS anomalies					
1970–73	12.2	8.4	6.5	13.9	9.6
1979	27.4	21.2	18.7	32.6	23.6
1980	30.7	20.7	18.5	29.1	23.1
Gastrointestinal					
Tracheoesophageal fistula					
1970–73	1.7	1.4	1.8	1.7	1.6
1979	1.8	1.8	1.5	2.1	1.7
1980	1.9	2.2	1.7	1.9	2.0
Rectal atresia stenosis					
1970–73	4.2	3.5	3.1	3.6	3.6
1979	3.8	2.9	2.9	2.9	3.1
1980	4.1	3.6	3.2	2.6	3.4
Genitourinary					
Renal agenesis					
1970–73	0.9	0.8	0.8	0.8	0.8
1979	1.0	1.3	1.0	1.5	1.2
1980	0.9	1.5	1.2	1.0	1.2
Hypospadias (rate per 10,000 male births)					
1970–73	45.5	42.7	38.4	41.3	42.2
1979	53.0	48.9	45.8	48.8	48.7
1980	58.7	53.8	45.8	44.8	50.8
Chromosomal					
Down's syndrome					
1970–73	9.7	8.3	6.6	8.9	8.3
1979	8.0	7.9	7.2	6.9	7.6
1980	8.7	7.4	5.7	8.6	7.3

Source: Centers for Disease Control, *Congenital Malformations Surveillance,* January–December 1979, issued December 1980; January–December 1980, issued February 1982.

Note: All congenital malformations—structural, biochemical, or chromosomal defects diagnosed at stillbirth or before one year of age in children whose parents resided in the metropolitan Atlanta area at the time of the infant's birth—1979: 39/1,000 (2/3 major malformations, 1/3 minor anomalies only). Nebraska birth defects surveillance—1979: 24/1,000 (85% major malformations). Florida congenital defects surveillance—1979: 18/1,000 (82% major malformations).

Table A.11 Frequency of Selected Reproductive Outcomes

Outcome	Frequency per 100	Unit
Azoospermia	1	Men
Birth weight < 2,500 g	7	Livebirths
Failure to conceive after one year of unprotected intercourse	10–15	Couples
Spontaneous abortion, 8–28 weeks of gestation	10–20	Pregnancies or women
Chromosomal anomaly among spontaneously aborted conceptions 8–28 weeks	30–40	Spontaneous abortions
Chromosomal anomalies among amniocentesis specimens to unselected women over 35 years	2	Amniocentesis specimens
Stillbirth	2–4	Stillbirths + livebirths
Birth defects	2–3	Livebirths
Chromosomal anomalies in livebirths	0.2	Livebirths
Neural tube defects	0.01–1	Livebirths + stillbirths
Severe mental retardation	0.4	Children to age 15 years

Source: Adapted from A. D. Bloom, ed., *Guidelines for Studies of Human Populations Exposed to Mutagenic and Reproductive Hazards* (White Plains, N.Y.: March of Dimes Birth Defects Foundation, 1981).

Table A.12   Major Malformations Common among Newborn Infants

Malformation	Rate per 1,000
Anencephaly	1.04
Myelomeningocele	0.33
Congenital hydrocephalus	0.36
Transposition of the great arteries	0.26
Ventricular septal defect	1.17
Hypoplastic left heart	0.23
Patent ductus arteriosus	0.72
Cleft palate	0.33
Cleft lip and cleft lip with cleft palate	0.78
Undescended testes	1.21
Hypospadias—first degree	2.12
Hypospadias—second or third degree	0.52
Clubfoot—all types	2.05
Talipes equinovarus	1.01
Metatarsus adductus	0.49
Calcaneovalgus	0.55
Congenital dislocation of the hip	0.78
Polydactyly—type B	2.15
Down's syndrome	1.53

Source: Adapted from A. D. Bloom, ed., *Guidelines for Studies of Human Populations Exposed to Mutagenic and Reproductive Hazards* (White Plains, N.Y.: March of Dimes Birth Defects Foundation, 1981).
Note: Prevalence of all major malformations is 26/1,000. These data are derived from surveillance of 30,681 infants of at least twenty weeks gestational age born at Boston Hospital for Women.

Table A.13   Sample Size of Comparison Groups Needed to Detect a
Certain-fold Increase with 95% Certainty over a Background
Frequency of 3, 7, or 15 Cases per 100 Events (Such as Births)

Frequency per 100	Sample Size of Comparison Groups	Increase In Frequency Detectable with 95% Power
3	50	7.7-fold
	100	5.3-fold
	250	3.3-fold
	300	3.2-fold
7	50	4.6-fold
	100	3.4-fold
	250	2.3-fold
	300	2.3-fold
15	50	3.0-fold
	100	2.4-fold
	250	1.8-fold
	300	1.7-fold

Source: Adapted from A. D. Bloom, ed., *Guidelines for Studies of Human Populations Exposed to Mutagenic and Reproductive Hazards* (White Plains, N.Y.: March of Dimes Birth Defects Foundation, 1981).

References Cited in Text
and Additional Suggested Reading

Bahn, Anita K. 1972. *Basic medical statistics.* New York: Grune and Stratton.

Barton, J., et al. 1981. Characteristics of respondents and non-respondents to a mailed questionnaire. *American Journal of Public Health* 70:308-11.

Bennett, A.E., and K. Ritchie. 1975. *Questionnaires in medicine: A guide to their design and use.* London: Oxford University Press.

Berdie, D.R., and J.F. Anderson. 1974. *Questionnaire: Design and use.* Metuchen, N.J.: Scarecrow Press.

Blomquist, H.K., K.H. Gustavson, and G. Holmgren. 1981. Mild mental retardation in children in a northern Swedish County. *Journal of Mental Deficiency Research* 25:169-86.

Bloom, A.D., ed. 1981. *Guidelines for studies of human populations exposed to mutagenic and reproductive hazards.* New York: March of Dimes Birth Defects Foundation, Medical Education Division.

Calabrese, E.J. 1978. *Pollutants and high risk groups.* New York: John Wiley.

Centers for Disease Control. 1980. *Congenital malformations survey, January–December 1979.* Washington, D.C.: U.S. Department of Health, Education, and Welfare.

Connors, D. 1960. *Community development: A guide to action.* Oakville, Ont.: Development Press.

Cook, J., and R. Wigley. 1975. *Community health: Concepts and issues.* New York: Van Nostrand.

Cowan, W.M. 1979. The development of the brain. *Scientific American* 241: 113-33.

Daugaard, J. 1981. *Symptoms and signs in occupational disease: A practical guide.* Copenhagen: Munksgaard, distributed by Year Book Medical Publishers, Chicago.

Davis, D.L., K. Bridbord, and M. Schneiderman. 1981. Estimating cancer causes: Problems in methodology, production and trends. In *Quantification of occupational cancer,* ed. R. Peto and M. Schneiderman, 285–316. Banbury Report 9. Cold Spring Harbor, N.Y.: Cold Spring Harbor Laboratory.

———. 1982. Cancer prevention: Assessing causes, exposures and recent trends in mortality for U.S. males, 1968–1978. *Teratogen, Carcinogen, and Mutagen* 2(2):105–35.

Dever, G.E. Alan. 1980. *Community health analysis: A holistic approach.* Germantown, Md.: Aspen System Corporation.

Doll, R., and R. Peto. 1981. The causes of cancer. *Journal of the National Cancer Institute* 66:1191–1308.

Doull, J.D., C.D. Klassen, and M.O. Amdur, eds. 1980. *Casarett and Doull's Toxicology.* 2d ed. New York: Macmillan.

Effrat, M. 1974. *The community: Approaches and applications.* New York: Free Press.

Ehrlich, Paul R., with Anne Ehrlich. 1968. *The Population bomb: The end of affluence.* New York: Ballantine Books.

Eifler, C.W., S.S. Stinnett, and P.A. Buffler. 1981. Simple models for community exposure from point sources of pollution. *Environmental Research* 25:139–46.

Epstein, S.S. 1978. *The politics of cancer.* San Francisco: Sierra Club Books.

Epstein, S.S., L.O. Brown, and C. Pope. 1982. *Hazardous waste in America.* San Francisco: Sierra Club Books.

Food Safety Council, Scientific Committee. 1980. *Proposed system for food safety assessment.* Washington, D.C.: Food Safety Council (1725 K Street, NW, Washington, D.C. 20006).

Functional model of health systems. 1971. Chicago: Aldine Atherton.

Gibbons, J.H. 1981. *Assessment of technologies for determining cancer risks from the environment.* Washington, D.C.: Office of Technology Assessment. Available from Superintendent of Documents, U.S. Government Printing Office, Washington, D.C. 20402.

Gifford, F.A. 1981. Estimating ground-level concentration patterns from isolated air-pollution sources: A brief summary. *Environmental Research* 25: 126–38.

Gittelsohn, A.M. 1982. On the distribution of underlying causes of death. *American Journal of Public Health* 72:133–40.

Green, L.W., and Anderson, C.L. 1982. *Community health.* 4th ed. Saint Louis: C.V. Mosby.

Green, L.W., M.W. Kreuter, S.G. Deeds, and K.B. Partridge. 1980. *Health education planning: A diagnostic approach.* Palo Alto, Calif.: Mayfield.

The Hammond Almanac. 1983. Maplewood, N.J.: Hammond Almanac, Inc.

Hart, F.C. 1978. Associates task IV—Economic analysis for Environmental Protection Agency. Contract 68014895, p. 6674, 12 October.

Hayes, W.J. 1975. *Toxicology of pesticides.* Baltimore: Williams and Wilkins.

Health Systems Agency of New York City. 1980. *Environmental and occupational health hazards primary care guide.* New York: Health Systems Agency.

Hook, E.B. 1981. Human teratogenic and mutagenic markers in monitoring around point sources of pollution. *Environmental Research* 25:178-203.

Howard, R. 1981. One man scoops the experts. In *These Times,* 18-31 March.

Hunter, D. 1978. *The diseases of occupations.* 6th ed. London: Hodder and Stoughton.

Infante, P.F., and M.S. Legator. 1980. *Proceedings of a workshop for assessing reproductive hazards in the workplace.* Washington, D.C.: Department of Health and Human Services. Available from the Superintendent of Documents, U.S. Government Printing Office, Washington, D.C. 20402.

Janerich, D.T., A.D. Stark, P. Greenwald, W.S. Burnitt, H.I. Jacobson, and J. McCusker. 1981. Increased leukemia, lymphoma and spontaneous abortion in western New York following a flood disaster. *Public Health Report* 96:350-56.

Juchau, M.R. 1981. *The biochemical basis of chemical teratogens.* New York: Elsevier/North-Holland.

Kallen, B., and J. Winberg. 1979. Dealing with suspicions of malformation frequency increase. *Acta Paediatrica Scandinavica Supplement* 275:66-74.

Karstadt, M., and R. Bobal. 1982. Availability of epidemiologic data on humans exposed to animal carcinogens. 2. Chemical uses and production volume. *Teratogenesis, Carcinogenesis, and Mutagenesis* 2(2):151-68.

Karstadt, M., R. Bobal, and I.J. Selikoff, 1981. A survey of availability of epidemiological data on humans exposed to animal carcinogens. In *Quantification of occupational cancer,* ed. R. Peto and M. Schneiderman, 223-42. Banbury Report 9. Cold Spring Harbor, N.Y.: Cold Spring Harbor Laboratory.

Key, Marcus, et al. 1977. *Occupational diseases: A guide to their recognition.* HEW (NIOSH) publication 77-181, rev. ed. Washington, D.C.: U.S. Department of Health, Education, and Welfare.

Landrigan, P.J., and E.L. Baker. 1981. Exposure of children to heavy metals from smelters: Epidemiology and toxic consequences. *Environmental Research* 25:204-24.

Landrigan, P.J., K.R. Wilcox, J. Silva, H.E.B. Humphrey, C. Kauffman, and C.W. Heath. 1979. Cohort study of Michigan residents exposed to polybrominated biphenyls: Epidemiologic and immunological findings. *Annals of the New York Academy of Sciences* 320:284-94.

Lebowitz, M.D. 1981. Respiratory indicators. *Environmental Research* 25:225-35.

Legator, M. S. 1979. Chronology of studies regarding toxicity of 1-2-dibromo-3-chloropropane. *Annals of the New York Academy of Sciences* 329:331-38.

Levine, A. 1982. *Love Canal: Science, politics, and people.* Lexington, Mass.: Lexington Books.

Levy, G. 1981. Pharmacokinetics of fetal and neonatal exposure to drugs. *Obstetrics and Gynecology* 58:9-16.

Lippman, M., and R. B. Schlesinger. 1979. *Chemical contamination in the human environment.* New York: Oxford University Press.

Longo, L. D. 1980. Environmental pollution and pregnancy: Risks and uncertainties for the fetus and infant. *American Journal of Obstetrics and Gynecology* 137:162-73.

Lowe, C. U. 1974. From the embryo through adolescence: Special susceptibility and exposure. *Pediatrics* 53:779-81.

Lyon, J. L., M. R. Klauber, W. Graff, and G. Chiu. 1981. Cancer clustering around point sources of pollution: Assessment by a case-control methodology. *Environmental Research* 25:29-34.

Mackarness, R. 1980. *Chemical victims.* London: Pan Books.

Mason, T. J., J. F. Fraumeni, R. Hoover, and W. J. Blot. 1981. *An atlas of mortality from selected diseases.* DHEW publication (NIH) 81-2397. Washington, D.C.: U.S. Department of Health, Education, and Welfare, National Cancer Institute, Division of Cancer Cause and Prevention.

Mason, T. J., F. W. McKay, R. Hoover, W. J. Blot, and J. F. Fraumeni. 1975a. *Atlas of cancer mortality among U.S. nonwhites: 1950-1969.* DHEW publication (NIH) 76-1204. Washington, D.C.: U.S. Department of Health, Education, and Welfare.

———. 1975b. *Atlas of cancer mortality for U.S. counties,* 1950-1969. DHEW publication (NIH) 75-780. Washington, D.C.: U.S. Department of Health, Education, and Welfare.

Matanoski, G. M., E. Landau, J. Tonascia, C. Lazar, E. A. Elliott, W. McEnroe, and K. King. 1981. Cancer mortality in an industrial area of Baltimore. *Environmental Research* 25:8-28.

Melton, L. J., D. D. Brian, and R. L. Williams. 1980. Urban-rural differential in breast cancer incidence and mortality in Olmsted County, Minnesota, 1935-1974. *International Journal of Epidemiology* 9:155-58.

Meyer, M. B., and J. Tonascia. 1981. Long-term effects of prenatal X-ray of human females. 2. Growth and development. *American Journal of Epidemiology* 114:317-26.

Miller, R. W. 1978. The discovery of human teratogens, carcinogens and mutagens: Lessons for the future. In *Chemical mutagens: Principles and methods for their detection,* vol. 5, ed. A. Hollaender and F. DeSerres. New York: Plenum Press.

National Commission of Community Health Services. 1966. *Health is a community affair.* Cambridge: Harvard University Press.

New York Academy of Sciences. 1977. *Cancer and the worker* (booklet). New York: New York Academy of Sciences (2 East 63rd Street, New York, New York 10021).

Oakley, G. T., Jr. 1975. The use of human abortuses in the search for teratogens. In *Methods for detection of environmental agents that produce congenital defects,* ed. T. H. Shepard, J. R. Miller, and M. Marois, pp. 189-96. New York: American Elsevier.

Paigen, B. 1982. Controversy at Love Canal. *Hastings Center Report,* June, p. 29.

Peters. J. M., S. Preston-Martin, and M. C. Yu. 1981. Brain tumors in children and occupational exposure of parents. *Science* 213:235-38.

Petitti, D. B., G. D. Friedman, and W. Kahn. 1981. Accuracy of information on smoking habits provided on self-administered research questionnaires. *American Journal of Public Health* 71:308-11.

Pless, J. B., and J. R. Miller. 1979. Apparent validity of alternative survey methods. *Journal of Community Health* 5:22-27.

Plunkett, E. R. 1977. *Occupational diseases: A syllabus of signs and symptoms.* Stamford, Conn.: Barrett Book Company.

Proctor, N. H., and J. P. Hughes. 1978. *Chemical hazards of the workplace.* Philadephia: J. B. Lippincott.

Quay, R., and P. Bowman. 1982. *A toxic waste handbook.* Galveston: Galveston County Toxic Waste Task Force.

Rea, W. J., D. W. Peters, R. E. Smiley, R. Edgar, M. Greenberg, and E. Fenyves. 1981. Recurrent environmentally-triggered thrombophlebitis: A five-year follow-up. *Annals of Allergy* 47:338-44.

Rinkus, S. J., and M. S. Legator. 1980. The need for both in vitro and in vivo systems in mutagenicity screening. In *Chemical mutagens,* ed. F. J. DeSerres and A. Hollaender, 6.365–473. New York. Plenum.

Roberts, D. W. 1982. Tissue burden of toxic pollutants. *Journal of the American Medical Association* 247:2142.

Roberts, H. 1979. *Community development: Learning in action.* Toronto: University of Toronto Press.

Segal, Edward, et al. 1980. *The toxic substances dilemma: A plan for citizen action.* Washington, D.C.: National Wildlife Federation.

Shephard, Roy J. 1982. *The risks of passive smoking.* New York: Oxford University Press.

Siemiatycki, J. 1970. A comparison of mail, telephone, and home interview strategies for household health surveys. *American Journal of Public Health* 69:238-44.

Sierra Club. 1981. *Training materials on toxic substances: Tools for effective action, books 1 and 2.* 2d ed. San Francisco: Sierra Club.

Sittig. M. 1980. *Priority toxic pollutants: Health impacts and allowable limits.* Park Ridge, N.J.: Noyes Data Corporation.

———. 1981. *Handbook of toxic and hazardous chemicals*. Park Ridge, N.J.: Noyes Publications.

Smolensky, J. 1977. *Principles of community health*. 4th ed. Philadelphia: W. B. Saunders.

Speth, G. 1980a. *Environmental quality, 1980*. Washington, D.C. Council on Environmental Quality. Available from Superintendent of Documents, U.S. Government Printing Office, Washington, D.C. 20402.

———. 1980b. *Toxic chemicals and public protection*. Washington, D.C.: Toxic Substances Strategy Committee. Available from Superintendent of Documents, U.S. Government Printing Office, Washington, D.C. 20402.

Stebbings, J. H. 1981. Epidemiology, public health and health surveillance around point sources of pollution. *Environmental Research* 25:1-7.

Stebbings, J. H., and G. L. Voelz. 1981. Morbidity and mortality in Los Alamos County, New Mexico. 1. Methodological issues and preliminary results. *Environmental Research* 25:86-105.

Stinnett, S. S., P. A. Buffler, and C. W. Eifler. 1981. A case-control method for assessing environmental risks from multiple industrial point sources. *Environmental Research* 25:62-74.

The susceptibility of the fetus and child to chemical pollutants. 1974. Proceedings of a meeting held in June 1973. *Pediatrics* 53, no. 5, part 2.

Suzuki, K. 1980. Special vulnerabilities of the developing nervous system to toxic substances. In *Experimental and clinical neurotoxicology*, ed. P. S. Spencer and H. H. Schaumburg. Baltimore: Williams and Wilkins.

Tokuhata, G. K., and M. W. Smith. 1981. History of health studies around nuclear facilities: A methodological consideration. *Environmental Research* 25:75-85.

Trieff, N. M., ed. 1980. *Handbook of toxic and hazardous chemicals*. Ann Arbor, Mich.: Ann Arbor Science Publishers.

United Auto Workers. 1981. *The case of the workplace killers: A manual for cancer detectives on the job*. Detroit: United Auto Workers.

U.S. Department of Health and Human Services. 1982. *The health consequences of smoking—cancer: A report of the surgeon general*. Publ. no. DHHS (PHS) 82-50179. Washington, D.C.: U.S. Government Printing Office.

———. 1975. *Basic concepts of environmental health* (booklet). HEW publication (NIH) 77-1254. Washington, D.C.: National Institute of Environmental Health Sciences (P.O. box 12233, Research Triangle Park, North Carolina 27709).

———. 1977. *Experiments in interviewing techniques*. NCHSR Research Report Series. HEW publication (HRA) 78-3204. Washington, D.C.: National Center for Health Services Research.

U.S. Department of Labor and Occupational Safety and Health Administration. 1979. *Lost in the workplace: Is there an occupational disease epidemic?* Washington, D.C.: U.S. Government Printing Office.

Vainio, H., M. Sorsa, and K. Hemminki, eds. 1981. *Occupational cancer and carcinogenesis.* Washington, D.C.: Hemisphere.

Waldbott, G. L. 1978. *Health effects of environmental pollutants.* 2d ed. Saint Louis: C. V. Mosby Company.

We're tired of being guinea pigs! A handbook for citizens on environmental health in Appalachia. 1980. New Market, Tenn.: Highlander Research and Education Center.

Wiese, W. H. 1981. Birth defects in areas of uranium mining. Paper presented at International Conference on Radiation Hazards in Mining. Colorado School of Mines, Golden, Colorado.

Wolff, M. S., H. A. Anderson, and I. J. Selikoff, 1982. Human tissue burdens of halogenated aromatic chemicals in Michigan. *Journal of the American Medical Association* 247:2112-16.

Wynn, M., and A. Wynn. 1981. Historical associations of congenital malformations. *International Journal of Environmental Studies* 17:7-12.

Zdenek, R. 1983. *Management essentials for community-based development organizations, neighborhood ideas.* Vol. 7, no. 9. Washington, D.C.: Civic Action Institute.

Contributors

Earon S. Davis
Ecological Illness Law Report
P. O. Box 1739
Evanston, Illinois 60204

Barbara L. Harper
Deparment of Preventive Medicine and Community Health
Division of Environmental Toxicology
University of Texas Medical Branch
Galveston, Texas 77550

Marvin S. Legator
Department of Preventive Medicine and Community Health
Division of Environmental Toxicology
University of Texas Medical Branch
Galveston, Texas 77550

Mary C. Lowery
Department of Preventive Medicine and Community Health
Division of Environmental Toxicology
University of Texas Medical Branch
Galveston, Texas 77550

Paul Mills
Department of Cancer Prevention
M. D. Anderson Hospital
6723 Bertner Street
Houston, Texas 77030

Michael J. Scott
Department of Preventive Medicine and Community Health
Division of Environmental Toxicology
University of Texas Medical Branch
Galveston, Texas 77550

Alice Shabecoff
30 Grafton Street
Chevy Chase, Maryland 20815

Ellen K. Silbergeld
Environmental Defense Fund
1525 18th Street N.W.
Washington, D.C. 20036

Kathleen Tiernan
School of Allied Health Sciences
University of Texas Medical Branch
Galveston, Texas 77550

William E. Townsley
Townsley, Griffin, and Bush
3550 Fannin Street
Beaumont, Texas 77701

Valerie A. Wilk
Farmworker Justice Fund
Migrant Legal Action Program
2001 S Street N.W.
Washington, D.C. 20006

Index

The Johns Hopkins University Press
The Health Detective's Handbook

This book was composed in Press Roman text and Times Roman display type by
A. W. Bennett, Inc., from a design by Chris L. Smith. It was printed on S. D. Warren's
50-lb. Sebago Eggshell paper and bound by the Maple Press Company.